Sleep Reset

The New Tools of Rest and Recovery

Natalie
Pennicotte-Collier

LONDON

Vermilion, an imprint of Ebury Publishing
20 Vauxhall Bridge Road
London SW1V 2SA

Vermilion is part of the Penguin Random House group of companies
whose addresses can be found at global.penguinrandomhouse.com

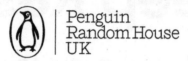

First published by Great Britain in 2024

www.penguin.co.uk

A CIP catalogue record for this book is available from the British Library

ISBN 9781785043987

The information in this book has been compiled as general guidance on
adult sleep. It is not a substitute and not to be relied on for medical advice.
So far as the author is aware the information given is correct and up to date
as of December 2023. Practice, laws and regulations all change, and the
reader is encouraged to obtain up-to-date professional advice on any such
issues. The author and publisher disclaim, as far as the law allows, any
liability arising directly or indirectly from the use or misuse of the
information contained in this book.

Typeset in 10.5/14.5pt Adobe Caslon Pro by Jouve (UK), Milton Keynes
Printed and bound in Great Britain by Clays Ltd, Elcograf S.p.A.

The authorised representative in the EEA is Penguin Random House Ireland,
Morrison Chambers, 32 Nassau Street, Dublin D02 YH68

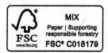

Dedicated to my insomnia: turning my nightmares into strength and the mission of my dreams.

CONTENTS

PREFACE

I had spent the night on the floor of the spinal injury unit in Great Ormond Street Hospital. I never thought I'd be so grateful to sleep on a thin foam mattress under bright hospital lights, all night long. My son Jude, aged 20 months, was in his cot bed beside me.

Some months before, Jude had become extremely poorly. We'd whisked him to A&E, where a brilliant consultant spotted what had been misdiagnosed at birth: Jude had a complex, rare spina bifida. His dad and I suddenly found ourselves faced with a shock diagnosis followed by a 12-hour complex spinal neurosurgery operation to release his delicate spinal cord, the powerhouse of his nervous system. After the operation, Jude looked as if he'd been bitten by a baby shark, with 200 raw stitches in his back.

The first sleepless week went by, with Jude's brilliant dad tag-teaming me and looking after our daughter, Darcy. These moments of crisis create enormous shock waves to our well-being and sleep health and Jude's operation led me to an incredibly intense period of insomnia, impacting me on every level. This stress after shock after stress after shock fragmented my sleep until it was at a bare minimum.

Insomnia corrupts your thinking, creating a true test of resilience. However, observing Jude's astonishing rate of healing, powered by sleep, showed me that sleep really is a superpower and, reflecting on that now, I can see how it became defining for me, fuelling a career pivot.

While Jude healed and slept, I needed to find respite from the onslaught of stress, rumination and catastrophising, and reconnect with my resilience. Spending time with world-class neurologists at Great Ormond Street gave me a fresh determination to learn all I could about the mind–body connection and the central nervous system. It also led me to the stunning realisation that I needed to take an integrated approach to my own sleep health, pushing me deeper into the understanding that sleep stress affects your entire day, and that holistic rest and recovery skills can transform your life.

Jude's determination to heal became a mirror for my own mindset – onwards and upwards; every moment a new possibility. I took a more holistic approach to help heal this intense chapter of insomnia and sought comfort and support in meditation and mindfulness. My recovery from insomnia became a strength, driving my mission. I resolved to devote my clinical professional career to supporting others with a laser focus on holistic sleep health.

Out of my family's desperate need, I had redefined my own well-being and wanted to bring this into all areas of my life and work. It pushed me into connecting with a bunch of incredible integrative GPs who knew of my work in the mental health community and with high-performance teen athletes. These GPs were acutely aware that there was very little they could offer the patients who came to them with insomnia and stress-related sleep issues, except for sleeping pills. We knew that together we could offer more.

And so I set up a sleep well-being clinic offering an entirely new holistic approach to sleep and insomnia, applying my training as a therapist supporting mental illness interventions in mindfulness-based cognitive therapy and clinical hypnotherapy.

Over the past decade, I have been on a personal mission to put sleep health centre stage. In my everyday work I help people understand their unique sleep and find sleep solutions that are both effective and sustainable. While sleep may be disrupted, challenged or stressed, it's never lost for good. When it changes, it's simply a signal that our sleep – and really, ourselves – needs kind-hearted compassion, care, support and focus.

With this book, I want to further extend that mission and help YOU take back control of your sleep health. Let's begin.

MINDFULNESS-BASED COGNITIVE THERAPY

The standard therapeutic approach for tackling sleep issues used by the NHS is cognitive behavioural therapy (CBT) for insomnia. It's helpful, but we know it doesn't work for everyone and people often approach me to enquire whether there's another way. And there is: over time, CBT evolved a new branch - mindfulness-based cognitive therapy, or MBCT - which encompasses the emerging science and wisdom of the body and breath in addition to standard CBT tools; I like to think of it as CBT plus.

MBCT goes further than CBT and trains the brain to stay in the here and now. It teaches you mindful skills: how to be mind-body aware, learning to orient your attention in helpful ways and accepting where you are as a sleeper. MBCT is an evidence-based framework for mental illness and stress-related challenges. A widely lauded treatment that's approved on the NHS for anxiety and depression, through my work and that of others it's now being recognised as highly effective for sleep problems too, and there are some brilliant new recovery tools based on MBCT in this book.

INTRODUCTION

Learning to sleep well is one of the single best things we can do to look after our physical and emotional well-being. Yet so many of us struggle to sleep well, and feel our energy and resilience erode as a result.

In my professional work supporting private clients, brands, elite sports organisations and schools, every day I hear, 'I am a terrible sleeper and I don't know what to do about it.' Despite the wealth of information out there on sleep hygiene and how to sleep well, we are still at a loss as to how to help ourselves and shift our sleep-stealing habits. Many of the people I work with have become experts at trying out sleep hygiene rules and other strategies, piling them on top of each other without a guiding mindset or a deeper understanding of the cause and effect of their habits, leading to short-term rather than long-lasting success. Simply being told what to do and what not to do without any consideration of how to implement new helpful behaviours with ease is not useful and, sadly, it's not working either.

Traditional sleep hygiene advice asks you to make changes to a list of habits. What I see when people are underslept and tired is that they don't know how best to make these changes. This book takes a deeper dive behind sleep hygiene and unlocks the tools you can use to support you in changing those habits.

Added to this, sleep science can be hard for tired minds to take in and the overwhelming amount of information out there doesn't help our exhaustion.

It's time for a sleep hygiene reboot, a modern update if you like, which will help you to uncover the unique and most effective strategies and routines that actually work for you.

SLEEP SCIENCE IS ENERGISING AND GUIDES US TO UNDERSTAND THAT SLEEP HEALTH STARTS FROM THE MOMENT YOU WAKE UP.

This book is different because I don't seek to judge or patronise. Instead, I trust in your inbuilt capacity for change. This is an open invitation to discover your ability to make changes, especially when times are challenging or you're tired of buying the latest sleep gadgets and surviving on ten coffees a day.

Instead of scaremongering, this book presents a new road map to help you understand, reset and protect your sleep health. I want to take the stress out of sleep with a sustainable, holistic method that shows you how you can rewire your approach to sleep, navigate your own sleep issues and formulate sustainable habits that you can draw on for life. I will show you how you can make clear and informed choices in how you think, behave and care for your mind and body.

Over the last few years, my method has needed to evolve to support people in making realistic change. This book was designed around what it feels like to do this work by yourself – with a tired mind – which means that the chapters might not follow your classic sleep hygiene or CBT for insomnia book.

Having been through various sleep challenges myself – from insomnia as a result of post-traumatic stress disorder, night terrors and nightmares, to undergoing neurosurgery for nerve damage, which led to disrupted sleep – I will sit on the same side of the pillow as you, encouraging consistent, gentle action directed towards building your sleep health for life.

And here's the best part: YOU are your own best sleep coach. With compassionate and positive action, you can make meaningful adaptations and gift yourself a good night's sleep.

THIS IS AN EASY-TO-FOLLOW, PRACTICAL AND
SUSTAINABLE APPROACH THAT YOU CAN
REALLY GET INTO BED WITH.

MY FIVE-WEEK SLEEP METHOD

This book was born out of my interactions with the people I meet
in my clinic and at my talks, workshops and school roadshows who
all ask the same questions:

- 'Where do I start?'
- 'How do I make changes to my sleep?'
- 'What can I learn?'
- 'How can I sleep better?'

You likely picked up this book because your sleep isn't working for
you. Or perhaps – and I hope this is the case – you are curious and
want to learn more about your sleep health in a practical, impactful
and accessible way. It's a universal truth that we tend to only reach
out when things are really bad, when we don't have the energy and
resources to challenge or change our thinking and behaviours. But
the power of sleep is the very foundation of well-being – it is the
first pillar – and it's something we should always be striving to
improve.

Sleep really is a stunning physiological support system that
resets us completely each and every night. It makes sense, therefore,
that we need a strong 360-degree approach to our sleep health.

It's almost certain that at some point in your life you have
experienced rubbish sleep, negative self-talk, self-doubt and have
maybe given up on meaningful goals in the past. The reality is that
our 24/7 life is addictive, distracting, busy and we are used to three-
second fixes. This is why sleep, at times, is so challenging – not
because you suck at sleep, life or habit change. Don't blame yourself
or assume you are getting things wrong.

Even though I don't know you yet, I know that you have three things that will help you meet any health goal:

1. You have self-talk and your breath.
2. You have a brilliant human brain – ready and hardwired to adapt and change.
3. You have a natural capacity to fail well at times and keep going.

I know this because everyone I have ever worked with has the exact same qualities, which drive helpful behaviour change and allow them to vastly improve their sleep within just a few weeks (not one hour or one day, but a few weeks). The tools and insight are all here for you if you choose to believe you can do it.

The integrative sleep method within this book draws heavily on research and a range of evidence-based practices that support sleep well-being – including circadian science, chronobiology, behaviour and habit change, breathwork, visualisation, mindfulness meditation and sleep hypnotherapy. These mind–body, non-medicated tools will support you in creating effective and lasting change. My Reset method also encompasses important new findings about the relationship between sleep, gut health and neurobiology.

The practical tools detailed throughout this book are designed to support your entire nervous system, allowing you to dial down sleep anxiety and a racing mind, helping to transform your sleep. They also work to enhance your mental health, helping to reduce stress, boost resilience and prevent burnout.

Combined, these changes will help you to develop a positive sleep well-being practice, so that you can achieve quality sleep night after night and regain calm, energy and focus in your daily life. This book is also something you can return to time and again if you feel that your sleep health is becoming problematic.

JUST AS YOU WOULD TWEAK, CHANGE AND
TRAIN TO OPTIMISE ANY OTHER ASPECT OF

YOUR HEALTH, IN FIVE WEEKS YOU CAN
PROTECT AND STRENGTH-TRAIN YOUR SLEEP
HEALTH IN A MEANINGFUL WAY, LEARNING
ZERO-COST, EVIDENCE-BASED TECHNIQUES
THAT WILL MAKE A REAL DIFFERENCE TO
YOUR SLEEP.

There have been many times in the past when stress, trauma, insomnia and disrupted sleep in the early hours of the morning have severely impacted the quality of my sleep, yet with the right tools and insight, I was able to get back up again. The mind–body approach in this book has changed my life for the better. It can do the same for you too.

YOU HAVE A CHOICE

It's useful to remember you always have a choice in how you respond to sleep struggles. All of the skills in this book are designed to help you build trust and confidence in your own ability to find a healthy sleep strategy that works for you, away from perfectionism or judgement. You get to choose to engage in whatever benefits *you* specifically.

MY GROUNDING PRINCIPLES

In my experience, there are some universal principles that help everybody look after their sleep health and, crucially, manage any sleep struggles. These principles underpin all of the tools you'll be learning throughout the book and I'd like to just touch on them now so you can get the most out of the Reset.

Core beliefs and mindset

Some of us are more sensitive to having our sleep disrupted. Life events such as financial stress, work pressures, family life and especially grief, illness and loss will always challenge and wobble our sleep. In short, sleeplessness is a natural part of life, but insomnia happens when we are too tired to update our thinking and coping habits and we get stuck.

Studies show that how we think about sleep affects our body's response, and therefore our actual sleep.[1] If we believe we're hopeless at sleep, this fuels unhelpful thinking and futile rumination, and early-hour catastrophising soon follows. Huge uncertainty, big questions and a racing mind about life's curveballs always seem to play out loudest in the early hours.

In Week 1 you'll focus on building a new, more positive mindset to reverse this downward spiral and enhance your sleep by redefining who you are as a sleeper and how you connect with this incredible asset.

Circadian science

The latest science makes it clear that harnessing the power and timing of light and darkness is the biggest single lever you have to transform your sleep health, focus and mental well-being.[2] In Week 2, you'll learn how your circadian rhythm works and the ways in which you can support it in order to enhance your sleep from the moment you wake up.

Self-compassion

Why does none of the sleep hygiene public health information mention the very thing that is needed for everyday sleep well-being and lasting habit change: self-kindness?

The ability to be self-kind is something we all have at our fingertips and yet underuse. However, it is what lies behind realistic habit change, powering so much of your sleep well-being.

I want to support you in being kinder to yourself and give you practical mind-coaching and audio tools (aka self-compassion) to help you reflect and uncover what's behind your stress-related insomnia, your racing mind, the busyness, the addictive tech habits . . . You need this missing component in your sleep toolkit to relearn the art of daily recovery.

> IT IS A FACT THAT SLEEP IMPROVES WHEN YOU ARE CARING, BRING A KIND FOCUS TO YOUR DAY AND TAKE SUPPORTIVE STEPS FORWARD.

Self-compassion is key to surviving life's natural turbulence and is essential for your Sleep Reset. It will lift your out of survival mode and allow you to grow into your sleep potential, safe in the knowledge that you can learn to let go of the toxic stressed sleep thinking that fuels shame and suffering. Self-compassion is a proven antidote to sleep shame and judgement.[3] Nothing is in your way – if you just choose to be nice to yourself on purpose.

In Week 3 we'll explore sleep-promoting nutrition, in Week 4 we will look at how self-compassion, gratitude and relearning essential breathing techniques can help you to combat sleep stress, and in Week 5 we will explore how rest, recovery and well-timed exercise are essential for our sleep health and well-being – all compassionate habits that will make a real difference to your sleep health.

Breathwork

Breathing is not just for oxygen; through neuroscience we can now demonstrate it is linked to brain function and behaviour, helping dial down mental stress and shift your state of mind.[4] Good breathing technique has also been shown to improve cardiovascular function during sleep in young, healthy individuals.[5]

From the moment we wake up and throughout our day, we experience subtle changes in alertness, energy and concentration, and our breathing changes to match this. Using the breathwork tools in this book will help you to control your breathing while also improving sleep quality, navigate feelings of tiredness and access self-compassion.

The breathwork tools operate on two levels: relearning functional breathing to help your sleep quality, and reimagining deliberate rest and recovery skills.

It's now undisputed that 'dysfunctional breathing' – a collective term for the way in which people breathe more rapidly through the mouth, holding tension in their jaw and shoulders, while breathing through just the upper part of their chest – is especially prevalent in sleep disturbances and insomnia.[6] However, the good news is that learning to support your breathing is one of the easiest things you can commit to as part of a daily Sleep Reset habit. You don't need any tech and, happily, it doesn't cost you a penny!

The breathing exercises in each week can be practised at any time, individually or in a sequence. They are also an effective way to create focus before using the hypnotherapy tools (see below). You can even wrap them around your teeth-cleaning routine, and they are also helpful to practise if you wake up during lighter stages of your sleep.

Sleep hypnosis

Clinical hypnotherapy changed my life in many ways that my younger, insomnia-challenged self could not even imagine. As a clinical hypnotherapist, sleep hypnosis is the cornerstone of my method and I see the resulting effects of behaviour change across all areas of my work. It really is the fastest way to experience lasting behaviour change and directly help your sleep well-being.[7]

I ask my clients to invest in creating a strong visualisation and mindfulness practice as part of their Sleep Reset, and, each week, I'm going to help you train your mindset with some highly effective hypnotherapy visualisations.

Sleep hypnosis, which involves the use of verbal suggestion and visual cues, helps you access deeper sleep and is also successful at treating insomnia and other sleep disorders including sleepwalking and sleep apnoea, as well as reducing midlife hot flushes and menopause sleep disturbances (see page 250).

There's no doubt that hypnosis has been misunderstood,

misrepresented and parodied in the past, but, happily, lifestyle medicine and the healing power of the mind are increasingly at the front and centre of sleep health, and the world's leading researchers are able to show for the first time through brain imaging exactly how beneficial hypnotherapy really is.

Dr David Spiegel, medical director of the Center for Integrative Medicine at Stanford University, and his colleagues used functional magnetic resonance imaging (fMRI) to identify the workings of the brain during hypnosis. They could see that a hypnotic state brings on enhanced concentration while actively dimming or dismissing other stimuli. Hypnotherapy enhances and increases the ability of the brain to control levels of relaxation.[8]

For many of my clients, it's comforting to know that self-hypnosis (which is also a form of visualisation) is like a powerful, wide-awake deep rest; indeed, people often describe it as feeling like bringing heightened attention to the things that matter to them. It enables them to concentrate on their inner world while still being fully in control and extremely aware of what is around them.

Neuroscience shows that self-hypnosis allows your brain to engage different circuits to enable behaviour change, build back sleep trust and activate better sleep quality.[9] Hypnotherapy for sleep can also alter and influence the way you process information in your brain and build up your confidence in sleep for life.

Over the last decade, people have become more aware of the undoubted benefits of mindfulness for mental well-being, but now we can also see what a perfect partner it is for our sleep struggles. In particular, mindfulness meditation is beneficial for sleep and can help significantly reduce the severity of insomnia and sleep latency (a fancy word for the time it takes for you to fall asleep), prolong total sleep time and, remarkably, even improve the depth and quality of our overall sleep.[10]

The sleep hypnosis tracks at the end of each week are simple but incredibly powerful and can be listened to at the start of the day, during the day or in the evening, depending on the exercise, and used as deliberate rest periods. They have different purposes depending on which week they sit in and will help you to reframe, step out of 'doing mode' (which we are all experts in) and take a moment to recharge in 'being' mode. The audio tracks can also allow us to sit with the things we can't change and find some resilient rest from stressors and the inevitable challenges life brings that often pressurise our sleep and erode our resting capabilities day and night.

The sleep hypnosis tools will help you feel empowered. Harnessing this valuable tool has helped my clients overcome challenges and enjoy enhanced sleep and mental health.

YOU CAN ACCESS THIS NATURAL MIND-BODY MEDICINE AT ANY TIME, IN ANY PLACE, TO CREATE PROFOUND CHANGES TO YOUR SLEEP HEALTH.

SLEEP STORIES

One of the most exciting and unique aspects of my work is that I get to listen to people just like you, who are perhaps curious about sleep health or have experienced poor sleep, and want to move past sleep stress and manage some of the challenging sleep problems that affect so many of us.

You'll find sleep stories throughout the book from people who, just like you, have struggled with their sleep. The good news is that all of them healed, found hope and a new way to access better sleep, rest and recovery. Their stories show what can happen when you commit to the Sleep Reset and take action to unlearn sleep-stealing habits and unhelpful thinking.

I also want to recognise the diversity of your sleep stories. We all have our own sleep stories, but there are some tried-and-tested steps we can all get on board with that will speak to our biology and make a difference.

HOW TO USE THE BOOK

Each week, I'll take you through a particular topic that, in my clinical work, I have seen can make a real difference to your sleep health. There are short, practical action points scattered throughout each chapter that encourage you to pause and take a moment to reflect on what immediate steps you can take to protect your sleep health. Then, at the end of each week, there are more extensive themed audio tracks, featuring sleep-changing hypnotherapy, Sleep Reset breathwork and visualisations to support you in making incremental changes and overhaul your attitude to sleep. These audio tracks are available at www.mindtonicsleep.com or via this QR code:

These tried-and-tested guided tools are highly effective and can be layered across the weeks. Besides guiding your personal sleep health journey, they will help you feel empowered, enable you to sleep deeper and teach you that habit-changing gem – self-kindness.

I want you to use this book in the same way I coach my clients: try to read through each chapter at the beginning of the week to understand the foundations of that week's focus, and then use the rest of the week to embed the tools and practices. It's these new habits and behaviours that can initiate your growing sleep potential. However, this book is for you, so feel free to take your time – it's normal and natural to go at your own pace; sleep needs patience at times. If you want to take two or three weeks for each week, please do. In this book you will be building a lasting new approach to *your* sleep health that is powered by you in your own time.

With this in mind, it's up to you whether you choose three, five or seven days of commitment each week to practise growing your new sleep health skills. You get to make your own rules based on what works for you. Find your own pace and take each week as you want or need to. Week by week, the tools can be layered up to build your *own* highly practical sleep health toolkit.

ACTION: HOW ARE YOU GOING TO USE THIS BOOK?

I'm so excited you're reading this book, but what I'm really excited about is how you're going to put it into action so that it sticks and becomes a jumping-off point for habit change, mental well-being and managing your stress.

Here's your first choice: How are you going to use this book? It may be that you love structure and want to go all-in and apply my advice verbatim. Or perhaps you prefer a more realistic lifestyle approach, something you can and will stick to. That might mean that from Sunday to Wednesday you choose to care for and focus on your sleep. Either approach is fine.

You'll find your own natural rhythm, but the real value is that in just five to ten minutes each day, you get to enjoy the lasting impact the tools have on the rest of your day and night.

THIS IS A HEALTHY DOSE OF REALISTIC SUPPORT TO FIND YOUR SLEEP SWEET SPOT.

This book has been designed to be your constant companion. You can make notes in it, flick through it and mark the pages and passages that resonate and that might be useful to refer to again in the days, weeks and months to come. You might also want to grab a notepad and pen to jot down your own notes, as well as have a device to hand so you can listen to the audio tools as you go along.

You deserve to build a sustainable approach to creating a rest and recovery strategy for any of the sleep issues that will arise at various times in your life. The tools laid out over the next five weeks will teach you how to wake up your sleep health and become aware of how best to give it a helping hand when you need it the most. They will give you confidence in your sleep, building trust and self-awareness to handle occasional disrupted sleep or full insomnia. Alternatively, if you want to protect your sleep health and put your mental health first, this is also the optimum way forward.

I meet all different versions of tired and wired, and the skills I'll introduce you to in this book have transformed the lives of many, including:

- An exhausted husband who was woken most nights by his young daughter, his wife who has Huntington's disease or his own overactive mind. As the breadwinner, he was desperate to manage his energy.
- A senior barrister who was having panic attacks and insomnia from his heavy workload.
- A mother whose child has many complex medical needs and who now finds she wakes at the slightest noise.
- An ultra-triathlete who needed to learn to sleep in the gaps between races.

If I could say one thing to you, it would be this: right now, in your hands, is an opportunity to optimise your mental and physical health through the power of sleep. Together we can redefine your unique relationship with sleep and lift you out of any sleep struggles. So let's wake up to sleep well-being, and get started.

REMEMBER, THE SLEEP RESET IS POWERED BY
YOU INVESTING SOME TIME IN WORKING
THROUGH EACH WEEK IN ORDER TO BUILD
YOUR SELF-INSIGHT AND SLEEP RESILIENCE,
HELPING YOU FORMULATE YOUR OWN
UNIQUE APPROACH TO SLEEP HEALTH.

WHEN TO SEEK EXTRA HELP

Don't be afraid to discuss significant changes in your sleep health with a sleep specialist professional or a behavioural sleep medicine therapist and coach. There is no doubt that having the opportunity to work one to one is helpful.

If after working through this book you are still experiencing chronic insomnia, it's essential that you seek one-to-one help from a medical professional (see also page 218).

Any further long-term sleep problems you may experience should be referred to your GP, using the insights and self-awareness you have gleaned from this book as a helpful reference point and account of your sleep journey so far.

BEFORE WE BEGIN

I see so many people in my clinics who don't understand how to sleep, and especially how to sleep well. Sleep is the most important pillar of well-being and, before we get started with Week 1 of the Reset, it's important to be knowledgeable about this powerful aspect of your health so you can support it with a practical, personal framework and strategy. However, I'm aware that some of you will just want to get stuck in, so feel free to skip over this chapter for now and perhaps revisit it once you've got some tools to improve your sleep health under your belt.

Healthy sleep is an emotional Band-Aid to modern life and the stress epidemic: good sleep is essential to good health. And yet the irony is that a lot of people feel so stressed about the quality of their sleep that this in turn impacts on sleep quality and waking hours, as well as fueling unhelpful habits.

We think we know the sleep basics, but then we try them and they don't work and we assume we can't sleep very well and develop performance anxiety. Then there's the quick-fix sleep aids. Perhaps your friends have told you about an amazing new supplement or sleep hack, and you've ended up taking it on an unfulfilling one-night stand. The internet is littered with well-meaning (often inaccurate) sleep tips and tricks, so-called 'bio hacks' that promise to optimise sleep. Newsflash: sleep doesn't need hacking; it needs science-based, wise attention.

Even when a change you try makes a difference, it's often not enough. Lavender, a warm bath and no tech just won't cut it. You still feel tired. There you are, still restless and wide awake for some or all of your nights.

Please don't despair. Help is on the way. Sleep can be so fragile, but like anything precious, when we pay it kind, committed and consistent attention, sleep will begin to strengthen in our favour.

LEARNING TO SLEEP AGAIN STARTS HERE.

SLEEP AND MENTAL HEALTH

Part of my mission is helping people understand the connection between sleep and mental health as they are so closely linked. However, I also appreciate this can be further fuel for your anxiety, so in this book I've chosen not to list out the negative aspects of not sleeping well. Instead, this book is about making sleep a priority in your life again and enabling you to get the sleep you deserve. However, if you would like to learn more and deep dive into the links between sleep and mental health, there is a section on my website about what happens when we don't choose to pay kind attention to our sleep: www.mindtonicsleep.com.

COMMON SLEEP MYTHS

Below are some common sleep myths I hear from my clients:

Myth: 'I'm too busy – proper sleep doesn't help me in day-to-day life.'

Fact: Sleep makes memories and enhances your capacity to learn. Sleep allows your brain to process and change through neuroplasticity (your brain's ability to rewire, adapt and change). This mostly takes place overnight in our sleep, helping us shape learning and memory and literally making it 'stick'. During sleep your brain helps you lay down deep learning and discard or consolidate all the information you acquired, read or heard during the day.[1]

Myth: 'My brain and body are fine on little sleep.'
Fact: Sleep gives the mind and body a five-star MOT. Sorry, but you're not exempt from Mother Nature's finest evolutionary design. It is rare for people to be able to sleep fewer than five hours a night without significant brain–body stress and damage.[2] A simple way to understand why *you* should care about great sleep is to look to sleep science. Overnight sleep allows the body to head into a full repair and upgrade – our personal MOT. It is also when we grow and when our muscles repair damage and recover from regular wear and tear inflicted throughout the day. Good sleep also plays a vital role in the function of our healthy immune response.[3] Only regular good sleep really allows these processes to work optimally for us.

Myth: 'I thought my brain was just dormant – literally offline – overnight.'
Facts: Far from it! Sleep is a really busy brain time and allows 'waste' to be cleared. While you sleep, your brain's housekeeping system, known as your 'glymphatic system', is working overtime in your brain and central nervous system. Like the perfect deep-clean shower, it refreshes, nourishes and cleans up the neurons and gets rid of the natural waste that accumulates in our waking hours, helping to replenish and renew your healthy brain.

Myth: 'Sleep feels like wasted time – I often sacrifice it to hit the gym late at night.'
Fact: Sleep can help you to meet your fitness goals in a smarter way. Sleep is the ultimate goal if you want to be stronger, smarter and focused. Only in sleep do we get physically

stronger. Our core body temperature drops, our blood pressure decreases and our breathing slows. Best of all, our central nervous system gets to rebalance and relax. Getting better sleep increases the likelihood of exercising and improving our muscle strength.[4]

Myth: 'I have good energy and power through – surely sleep isn't that important.'
Fact: Sleep helps us stay strong and energised. Sleep keeps your metabolism healthy and regulates appetite. Addressing your sleep can help tackle issues with your blood sugar, including your risk of diabetes and heart disease.[5] Did you know that sleep also plays a vital role in supporting your heart health? Good sleep helps to keep cardiovascular problems at bay and also aids us in maintaining healthy levels of cholesterol.[6]

GETTING INTO BED WITH BETTER SLEEP QUALITY

'Sleep quality' is a term that helpfully describes how restful and deeply restorative sleep is. Sleep time and quality both really matter.
Sleep quality:

- helps YOU understand your overall sleep health beyond just how many hours you've slept
- is something you can helpfully gain control of with your daily habits and the Sleep Reset
- is not forced and occurs naturally without too much striving or stressing

Good-quality sleep generally makes us feel energised and refreshed within the first hour of waking up, and helps power us through our day with energy, focus and without relying too much on afternoon caffeine crutches or excessive napping.

It's useful to note that if we crash out like a light on the sofa or as soon as our head hits the pillow, it's often because we are chronically underslept or excessively sleepy.

As sleep is so often misunderstood, it can be useful to strip it back and remind yourself what healthy sleep looks like.

Falling asleep (sleep onset):

- 'Realistically, I can fall asleep within 5–30 minutes without any stress.'
- 'I notice I regularly feel sleepy at a similar time of night.'
- 'I trust in my familiar bedtime routine and accept I may wake fleetingly or move in the night, which is normal.' (Being awake at times is part of normal, healthy sleep!)

Sleep continuity:

- 'I frequently hit my sleep target for adults: 7–9 hours per night.'
- 'The time I spend in bed actually asleep is around 80 per cent.'
- 'I experience infrequent wake-ups in the night and trust I will fall asleep again.'*
- 'I regularly sleep well throughout the night.'

Sleep timing:

- 'I wake up mostly refreshed and notice this happens automatically, even at weekends.'
- 'I feel energised within an hour of waking up.'
- 'I don't suddenly fall asleep during the day and I feel natural peak energy and rest points.'
- 'I am not reaching for emergency long naps in the day.'

---

* It's natural and normal to have wake-ups in the night. As a general guide, if you're experiencing more than four or five wake-ups, your sleep needs support.

When we are in good sleep health, the everyday habit of waking up each morning and falling asleep feels somewhat effortless. Falling asleep feels easy and sleep turns into something that most of us take for granted ... until things go awry and/or we experience sleep stress that can turn into broken and inadequate sleep.

HIDDEN SIGNS OF POOR SLEEP QUALITY

- excessive daytime sleepiness
- needing caffeine to get by
- poor focus and brain fog
- shortness of breath
- tendency to drift off easily
- feeling moody
- eyes stinging
- struggling in the afternoon at work
- taking long naps
- yawning all afternoon
- falling asleep on the commute

These are all common signals that you may need more sleep. If you can relate, it's really worth committing to the Sleep Reset for the next five weeks.

NATURAL SLEEP TURBULENCE

We all have reasons for being awake when we'd like to be asleep. Perhaps yours are outside noise, a snoring partner, a needy pet, a new shift schedule or hormonal changes. I know I am not the only person whose sleep has been fragmented by health anxieties, loss, fears or a million other complex reasons – in other words, the full catastrophe of life.

'Sleep turbulence' is the way I describe the sleep disturbances I see every week that are widely underreported as they don't yet meet the criteria of a sleep disorder or insomnia, and it's a term we'll revisit throughout the book. I have chosen not to focus solely on insomnia as I know many of you will be coming to this book with sleep struggles and sleep deprivation. Sleep deprivation is a little like inebriation: the worse it is, the hazier our judgement of how much sleep we actually had.

Some of the most common 'accidental' insomnia-fuelling factors that I regularly see are:

- Feeling unsure of how to prioritise managing our stress and not setting boundaries in our life.
- Unresolved stress from putting things off, creating further stress in the mind.
- A racing mind fuelled by the 'always on' lifestyle of doing too much without scheduled rest, spiking cortisol all day.
- Consumption habits replacing stress-coping strategies, with caffeinated days leading to night-time alcohol consumption while staying up late scrolling on mobile phones, watching TV or gaming.
- Self-defeating thoughts, beliefs and disaster-thinking loops where we wake in the night frequently and then worry that we may have insomnia and struggle to imagine sleep will return again.
- Trying too hard to get to sleep, which can have the opposite effect.
- Unrealistic expectations about the amount of sleep we should be getting.

There will also be moments in life when inevitable sleep challenges arise. You are not alone! Recent studies have found that as much as 30–50 per cent of the general population experiences sleep problems.[7]

Sleep difficulties are particularly common in women, children and those over 65. In fact, roughly half of the elderly population complains of insomnia.[8] Therefore, to have trouble sleeping at some point in your life is quite normal.

There are a number of reasons why sleep problems can develop:

- Effects of ageing: when people get older they tend to sleep less deeply and may also sleep less well at night. Sometimes people will then tend to drop off to sleep during the day, which again reduces the need for sleep at night. This in itself is not a problem, but often not sleeping at night becomes a great cause for worry, frustration and concern, which in turn leads to sleeping less well.
- Excessive need to go to the toilet at night, known as nocturia: most common in adults over the age of 50, although can occur at any age. It refers to a regular frequent need to wake up and urinate during sleep.[9] This can also happen for other reasons of course, such as pregnancy. Getting out of bed at night isn't always a huge problem but can be frustrating if you find it difficult to get back to sleep.
- Perimenopause and menopause: many women report disturbed sleep around the peri- and menopause, often related to hot flushes. Difficulty sleeping often remains and, generally, post-menopausal women are less satisfied with their sleep, with as many as 61 per cent reporting insomnia symptoms (we'll explore hormonal changes in women further on pages 247–254).[10]
- Chronic pain: this again can be more common in older age with joint problems such as arthritis.
- Medication: some medicines can interfere with sleep, so it is worth checking with your doctor if you are on any tablets.
- Obstructive sleep apnoea: this is a very treatable condition present in around 5 per cent of both genders. Although most common in middle age, some research points to this affecting

as many as one in eight – though the figure is likely to be higher (see page 222 for more on this condition).[11]

- Restless legs syndrome (RLS): this is present in about 5 per cent of the population.[12] People with RLS have an urge to move their legs and find it really hard to keep their legs still. This often comes later in life and can also be made worse by some medicines as well as pregnancy.

- Stress, worry and anxiety: when someone is stressed and anxious they may often find it hard to get off to sleep, with their mind full of worries and their body tense (we'll explore this further in Week 4).

- Depression and low mood: disturbed sleep is a common symptom of depression. It is quite usual for depression to lead to early-morning waking and an inability to get back to sleep, or alternatively to having difficulty getting off to sleep.

- Bereavement trauma and loss: the emotional upset of bereavement or other trauma can affect sleep. Nightmares and upsetting memories are common.

- Environment: our surroundings can make a big difference to how we sleep. For example, a bedroom that is overly hot or overly cold, a bed that is too hard or too soft, a room that is too noisy or too light can all make a difference to how well someone sleeps (see page 28 for tips on optimising your sleep environment). Sleeping in a strange place can also affect someone's sleep.

- Disrupted sleep routine: people who work shifts that change frequently often have disrupted sleep (see page 235 for more on shift work). This gets worse with age and is affected by lifestyle factors such as smoking and drinking alcohol.

When sleep goes awry, it can play on your mind, distract you and snatch at your energy and resilience. You can get stuck in the same habit loop and feel hopeless, lacking the energy and resources to fix it. But it needn't be this way. Sleep turbulence is a natural part of life, not a battle to be fought or won. The only 'win' is exercising more choice in how best to care for and respond to your sleep. By choosing to pay kind, healthy attention to your relationship with sleep, you can cope with sleep turbulence. It is possible, at any stage in life, to learn and develop the skill of sleeping well at night. In fact, it is essential.

ACTION: IDENTIFY YOUR SLEEP RESET MOTIVATION

It's incredibly valuable to your Sleep Reset to focus on one or two good reasons why you will start to look after your sleep health in order to improve your mental health. It's worth thinking about this and writing down your reasons, because getting really clear on what being well slept will mean for you will help you move beyond initial motivation and guide your focus.

Think about why you want to invest time in your sleep.

- What are the things you really want to gain?

- How will you know when you reconnect to your sleep health?

Think about how you will benefit. I've talked about some of the benefits, but you'll have personal reasons too. Start with this sentence stem:

'Better sleep will . . .'

_____

_____

People often write things like:

- give me back my energy and life

- make me feel I am prioritising my health

- balance my mood so that I feel more present

- help me manage chronic pain

- fuel me to reach my athletic goals

- bring me more energy during the day to move

- reduce anxious thoughts

- put my mind at ease and balance my energy and recovery

- give me better focus

- stop me snapping at my family

- gift me my social life back

- enable me to show up for my partner and loved ones more

BE OPEN AND TRY SOMETHING
DIFFERENT, BECAUSE WHAT YOU HAVE DONE
BEFORE IS PROBABLY NOT USEFUL OR
SUPPORTIVE.

BEDROOM BASICS

Before we get started with building your sleep mindset in Week 1, there's an easy Sleep Reset tool you can use straightaway: optimising your sleep space.

You may already be familiar with some of the advice in this section, but upgrading your sleep environment is an easy win for optimising your sleep health. Choose one or two things you can do straightaway and revisit this section as and when you need a lift – sometimes it's the little things that can make such a difference.

Your bed

Your bed is the most important piece of furniture in your home! For me, it is the number one sleep health purchase. When it's time to update your bed, whether you go for a bed frame or a divan base, ensure it provides good support. Look for sturdy, high-quality bed frames that are within your budget. For a queen- or king-size bed, make sure your frame has a strong centre support that will prevent the mattress from bowing.

Choosing the best mattress

Making an uninformed choice when choosing a new mattress can lead to problems in the future including back or shoulder pain, which in turn can lead to sleep deprivation, poor sleep quality and even having to go mattress shopping again sooner than you'd like (which is bad for your wallet and the planet!).

NOT SURE WHEN TO REPLACE YOUR MATTRESS?

Look for dipping in the middle, worn fabric and squeaky springs as well as signs of discomfort.

Natural materials such as wool and cotton are perfect for mattresses (and indeed bedding) as they are breathable, wick moisture away from the skin and help regulate body temperature. Aside from comfort and great support, temperature regulation is absolutely key (see below). Great sleep is highly sensitive to subtle changes in temperature so this really matters for your sleep wellbeing. The reality is that our beautiful inner sleep system is fussy! It works best in overnight, dark, cool conditions. If you get too hot, it will lead to fragmented sleep and you'll wake up more easily. In addition, many sleep-related neurons in the brain are highly temperature sensitive. Natural fibres can also help to control dust and stay clean and dry for longer, which can help if you suffer from allergies or asthma.

It's also important to look for top-to-toe comfort and support in your mattress. This is really key as we often share our beds and naturally shift positions at least 20 times each night.

GO FOR A TEST DRIVE

Once you've found a few mattresses you're interested in, try them out if you can. Remember that your mattress needs to be comfortable for an entire night, not just a few minutes. Simulate sleeping by removing your coat and shoes, grabbing a pillow and lying down in your normal sleeping position for at least ten minutes. This should be just enough time for your body to comfortably relax and get a real feel for the mattress.

Room temperature

Many studies have shown that your bedroom temperature has a big impact on sleep well-being, and maintaining a cool body temperature at night can help you sleep longer.[13] Generally, we want to be in what we call a 'thermal neutral zone', which is on the slightly cooler side. Ideally, to initiate sleep, the temperature of your sleep space should be around 16–18°C max all year round. But I know that, in reality, this is difficult to control, so don't get too hung up on this. What catches a lot of people out in the cooler months is cranking up their central heating without realising the subtle impact this has on their sleep quality, so try to bear this in mind. During a heatwave or warmer weather, you can help cool your room by drawing the curtains or closing the blinds during the day.

As we'll see in Week 2 (page 64), a drop in body temperature is associated with sleep onset. We can facilitate this by creating a cool sleeping environment as much as possible.

Pillow talk

Pillows are an easy, low-cost update and are vitally important for neck support. A key ally to help combat the 'skeletal tech neck' (caused by spending too much time in 'digital scrolling position' with your head tilted far forward) that is on the rise in our hyper-tech generation, they also support good postural breathing.

There are lots of new pillows on the scene:

- Organic wool: the greenest of the green when it comes to filling. Made up of small balls that can be teased out to produce a customised level of fluff, wool-fill pillows are not resource intensive and are very long-lasting.
- Tencel: a great vegan alternative to wool, Tencel is made from raw natural fibres derived from eucalyptus grown in sustainable forests. Even more eco-friendly than bamboo, it's low energy and uses chemicals that are environmentally sensitive.
- Feather: feather pillows offer softness and support. The feathers used in a quality pillow are very small and highly curled. They are nature's natural spring.
- Down: if you want the softest, gentlest pillow, go for down. Down comes from a bird's fluffy undercoat – think feathers without quills. Down pillows are soft, puffy and supple, known as the ultimate luxury, but are not meant to provide support.
- Microfibre (synthetic alternative to down): this is just as soft and luxurious but better suited to people who don't want to use animal products or who suffer from allergies.
- Memory foam: memory foam comes with its own issues and is not biodegradable. These pillows remember your sleep contour all night long. You stay comfortable because the pillow adjusts to your individual shape, which allows your shoulders, neck and head to rest in a natural position.
- Buckwheat: looking for something all-natural and plant-based? Buckwheat pillows are filled with husks from buckwheat seeds. They offer hard support.

There are also orthopaedic neck pillows, body pillows, lumbar pillows and wedge pillows that can help with everything from lower back support and joint pain to headaches and acid reflux.

If you sleep on your stomach, you may need a soft pillow that keeps your head closer to the mattress, maintaining the integrity of your neck's natural alignment. Back sleepers should opt for a firmer, flatter pillow to keep the head and neck in alignment. A pillow placed under your stomach and pelvis may help to prevent back pain.

GETTING THE RIGHT PILLOW IS A GREAT WAY TO INVEST IN YOUR BEST REST, ACTING AS A CUE FOR A GREAT NIGHT'S SLEEP. IT'S A SURPRISINGLY SIMPLE, LOW-COST PSYCHOLOGICAL BOOST THAT WORKS REALLY WELL.

WHAT ABOUT ALLERGIES?

Allergy flare-ups aren't generally caused by the pillow fill itself, but by the dust mites that make their home in - particularly natural-fill - pillows. To reduce allergens, invest in a pillow protector, air your pillows out now and again, plump them up regularly, beating out any dust and mites, and, where suitable, wash the pillow every six months, but check the manufacturer instructions.

Bring the outside in

It's widely known that spending time outdoors is good for your health. Exposure to nature can reduce stress levels, boost your immune system and even lower blood pressure. But how do we bring this feel-good factor into the bedroom to encourage a good night's sleep?

Biophilic design uses features or patterns that elicit a similar mental and physical response to those we have when we're in nature.[14] A sleep space designed with biophilic features will create a calm atmosphere for us to unwind in:

- Bedding should be natural and breathable: cotton and linen are perfect for a biophilic scheme.
- Surround yourself with nature by bringing greenery like house plants into your room.

- When and if you can, open a safe window. Research has shown that both sleep quality and next-day performance can be improved by increasing the amount of clean outdoor air within the bedroom.[15] When measured, sleep quality and the freshness of bedroom air improved significantly when the CO_2 level was lower.

ACTION: SLEEP SPACE UPGRADE

In my experience, some people love to know how to create the 'perfect' room, while others just want to know the small things they can do, grounded in science, that make a difference.

Thinking about what you have read in the section above, what capacity do you have, right now - without putting any pressure on your sleep - to freshen up your sleep space? What prompts you to think, *This is an easy win for me*? Think: *Is it possible? Is it kind? Is it doable? Is it realistic?* As always, it comes down to choice.

- What tiny tweaks or upgrades can you make in your sleep space?

- What are you inspired to do right away?

- What is one thing that has sparked that rest-easy feeling in you?

If you are looking for seductive promises of fast overnight sleep-perfecting fixes, I'm afraid you won't find them here. There's a very clear reason that I share a guide across five weeks and that's because, over the years, I've seen that this period is effective and sustainable. It provides enough time for your inner sleep coach to kick in and for you to embed these skills into autopilot, helping to lift you out of insomnia or sleep turbulence and into sleep health. This is not a quick fix and it will feel much slower than you're used to – but that's what drives lasting change.

There's an oft-repeated cliché in sleep books that a good sleeper is someone who does nothing in order to sleep well. We all want our sleep to be easy and automatic, take care of itself and feel less of a struggle, but the truth is that, if you look at the rhythm of a good sleeper's day, there are things such as stress management, good nutrition and good physical and mental well-being in the background that all support their sleep health.

When you complete the steps in this book, it will feel effortless and like you're doing 'nothing' just before you go to sleep, even though your sleep health is always working behind the scenes. And, much like with the Olympic and elite athlete squads I work with as a performance well-being coach, lasting success is in the learning, developing resilience and self-awareness along the way.

You're going to become a sleeper who connects with the value in *all* of your sleep (even the nights when you only manage a few hours), spending time learning new tools to adapt your potential for rest and recovery. When you do this, sleep can become your most valuable health asset, giving you energy and a feeling of control over your own life.

Instead of fixating on fixing your sleep, you're going to get curious about your personal sleep health, learn to understand it and find out what works for YOU, the unique sleeper. This will be different for everyone: your sleep health is as individual and beautifully complex as your body and mind. You'll start with small changes, then layer them for maximum results. And crucially, by the end of this book, you'll know what works for you and have your own blueprint for sleep health.

All the tools and actions in this book should help you to shake off any sleep-stealing habits, deal with times of sleep turbulence and protect your sleep health, starting with developing a sleep health mindset with compassion at its core – Week 1 – as the first powerful step towards a meaningful and lasting approach to recovery and thriving in life.

Welcome to your journey to healthy sleep!

WEEK 1: BUILDING YOUR SLEEP MINDSET

Welcome to Week 1 of your Sleep Reset! In this first week, whether you are brand new to working on your sleep or are in sleep SOS, we will be looking at your sleep mindset, uncovering how you feel about sleep and your current sleep health, and focusing on rewiring your mind in order to step away from autopilot thinking and let go of old thinking habits that are holding back your sleep potential. This week you'll build some strong foundational principles that are low effort but will give you a big return on investment.

Try to connect with the actions this week away from a judging mind and without expectation. The tools at the end of this chapter (page 54) will help you to generate more helpful thoughts, especially around your sleep and recovery.

YOUR SLEEP HEALTH MINDSET MATTERS

I have found over the years that sleep is one of the most misjudged and misunderstood parts of our daily experience. I want to change that for you. But first, I want you to think about what sleep means to *you*.

Everyone has their own unique way of describing what poor sleep means to them, both how it feels and how they handle it. It's natural that we use this self-critical language on autopilot, but it's the opposite of useful. It's an ineffective and tiring way of keeping us stuck in a cycle of rumination with a cascade of physiological stress.

RESEARCH TELLS US THAT THE QUALITY OF
OUR THINKING BECOMES MORE NEGATIVE
WHEN WE ARE UNDERSLEPT.[1]

As a sleep therapist, the first thing I do with my clients is take all
the pressure off and share the 'sleep paradox': the harder we force or
look for quick hacks/fixes, the more we stress sleep health and find
it more challenging and elusive. The mind–body connection is
really powerful – when we throw off stress chemicals, it upsets our
sleep–wake rhythm. How you think and feel about sleep has a
powerful effect on that rhythm.

'THE TOTAL EFFECT OF ANYTHING IS A
COMBINED PRODUCT OF WHAT YOU THINK
YOU ARE DOING AND WHAT YOU THINK
ABOUT WHAT YOU ARE DOING.'

DR ALIA CRUM, ASSOCIATE PROFESSOR OF
PSYCHOLOGY AT STANFORD UNIVERSITY AND
DIRECTOR OF THE STANFORD MIND &
BODY LAB[2]

It may surprise you to learn how much your beliefs and your thoughts
about sleep really matter – they have a physiological effect. They
directly impact what's going on on the inside. Evidence shows that
your mindset has a massive impact on your stress and on how you
sleep, which is why setting a really healthy Sleep Reset commitment is the first action for this week.[3]

ACTION: **YOUR SLEEP RESET COMMITMENT**

This is an effective way to commit to the process of looking after
your sleep health. Setting an intention will help you to navigate
away from judgement and perfectionism traps, refocus your

thoughts and feelings in a helpful way and avoid the sleep paradox I mentioned above.

This commitment is inspired by research around how self-compassion underpins healthy sleep and helps reframe your Sleep Reset journey to build success across the weeks.[4] Here the focus is your sleep health, but this commitment tool also works incredibly well for other habits/health goals or times when you want to change.

Please try not to skip this part – it matters. YOU matter. Taking a moment to 'think in ink' now will be a really useful support for you across the Reset. However, if this feels too difficult right now, you can return to this in the coming weeks.

Follow the steps below to write your own Sleep Reset commitment:

Dear Me,

Step 1: Show awareness of your struggle or lack of focus on your sleep well-being.

Acknowledge that this is hard and maybe something you have avoided attending to.

For example:

'I am fully committing to focus on my sleep health this month because it matters, I matter and I am sleep-deprived.'

'This has been something I've found challenging. I can sense my discomfort and struggle.'

'Argh, I know my sleep has been ignored and doesn't feel great – it needs a reset.'

Step 2: Remind yourself of a time you overcame adversity.

You might already have a PhD in coping with a bad night's sleep and dealing with stress and self-doubt at some stage in your life. Now, take a moment to think about your toughest night's sleep; maybe this was just one night for you or maybe it was a longer episode of really poor sleep. Describe how you showed up for yourself during that period and coped the following day.

For example:

'I know I can do hard things. I have suffered and survived bad sleep. I can make this easier for myself just by showing up and actually doing the tools.'

'I place trust in myself to do this because . . .'

'No matter what, I deserve to care for myself to focus on my sleep health and I will complete this five-week Reset.'

Step 3: What would you say to a trusted, well-loved, well-regarded friend if they were struggling?

Show yourself the same empathy and encouragement for the journey ahead.

For example:

'Like a friend I will show up - not judge - and accept the journey's highs and hurdles along the way.'

'I commit to being kind and dedicated. I will be my own ally and not sabotage sleep with poor choices or habits that are holding me back.'

'It's okay to keep going.'

Step 4: Understand the universal truth - you are not alone.

What's universally true is that our sleep changes across our lifespan and the majority of us will experience sleep struggles. Each night is often utterly unique and different from the last, even if the hours are the same. Take a moment now to write down a statement that acknowledges this. I find it helpful to keep this in my phone or journal as a reminder for those times when I might not have had the sleep I wanted.

For example:

'Sleep is not always perfect; I know that. I am learning to care for my sleep and I acknowledge I am not alone in experiencing sleep stress, but I am also not alone in being born able to sleep.'

'Sleep is in my biological blueprint and I can find a way to help protect and care for my sleep.'

Step 5: Write a kind coaching statement to yourself.

Make a final commitment to your goal.

For example:

'There is no "failure", only learning, and I've got this.'

'I am learning to sleep well once again. I will turn this sleep guide into positive action - and I won't regret it.'

'I can improve my sleep health for the long term. Sleep health is my goal.'

Sometimes you and sleep will get along easily, but when life gets in the way, you may disconnect for a while and seem to fall out. Sometimes it will need focus, at other times it will feel effortless.

I'd like you to see yourself as having a lifelong connection and relationship with sleep. Rather than battling with it, view it as a long and fruitful partnership for life. Just like an authentic partnership, when this relationship goes awry, it can play on your mind, steal your focus and reduce your energy and resilience. By choosing to pay kind, healthy attention to your relationship with sleep, you can cope with sleep turbulence, step away from unhelpful thinking and notice an improvement in the quality of your sleep.

UNDERSTANDING YOUR SLEEP HEALTH MINDSET

Your sleep story

I call our past experiences of sleep our 'sleep story'. Like mine, your sleep story will be made up of all the episodes in your past – the good as well as the challenging.

Your sleep cannot be perfect or exactly the same every night of your life. I see time and time again how the myth of a perfect 'eight hours' sleep or else' actually steals sleep and creates sleep anxiety. You get to choose where to shine your focus and attention in order to enhance your relationship with sleep rather than simply obsessing about how many hours you got last night and being your own worst critic.

Every week I also work with people who hanker after a sleep expectation from the past: 'I used to sleep for eight hours a few years ago.' Even if they are now regularly having around seven hours' sleep per night, this past perceived perfection itself becomes a barrier.

Striving for sleep perfection or having an attachment to a sleep ideal is responsible for so much wasted precious sleep each night and worry about the consequences of sleeplessness. It's essential that you reframe and release those comparison thoughts and instead meet your sleep exactly where it is this week. Begin by believing in and building that healthy self-awareness and mindset that will help strengthen your sleep health.

ACTION: THINK ABOUT YOUR OWN SLEEP STORY

- What is your current sleep story?

- Do you think you are striving for unrealistic sleep perfection?

- Has it always been this way? If not, when did it change?

- What is your expectation of healthy sleep?

Understanding yourself as a unique sleeper is crucial to resetting good sleep health.

Sleeping in cycles

In 2017, fellow sleep evangelist Nick Littlehales, who pioneered the idea that sleep is one of the most important factors in sporting success, invited me to his roadshow to share my mind–body techniques for performance sleep. We had both dedicated our careers to helping people take sleep seriously and waking everyone up to rest and recovery as a core foundation to sleep health.

One really useful tool that we both shared in our approach was thinking about having five full sleep cycles each night as opposed to seven to eight hours' sleep. This is a realistic way to be proactive with your sleep across the week. If your aim is to sleep well, but your week is mixed with early and late nights, the strategy to aim for 35 sleep cycles across the week gives you a helping hand to plan for and schedule in good sleep.

For me, thinking about sleeping in cycles instead of a more judgemental view of how many hours' sleep you've had per night is a helpful, realistic way to boost everyone's sleep health, but is especially beneficial for shift workers, frontline staff and, of course, new parents. I'm so pleased that Nick brought this new definition of sleep and recovery into the mainstream. Take a look at the action below – could you try it this week and see if this mindset shift is helpful for you?

ACTION: AIM FOR 35 SLEEP CYCLES PER WEEK

This week, aim to shift your mindset to thinking about how many sleep cycles you've had per night to help you work out your ideal bedtime and manage sleep across your week.

- Step 1: Choose your morning wake-up time.

- Step 2: To work out your ideal bedtime, aim for five full 90-minute sleep cycles each night and count backwards from there.

- Step 3: Allow for an additional 20 minutes of phasing into sleep.

For example, if your wake-up time is 6am, aiming for five sleep cycles of 90 minutes will guide you to a bedtime of around 10pm.

Of course, life often gets in the way and things need to be flexible. If you have to have a later bedtime and only experience four full sleep cycles, you can build that 90-minute lost cycle into your next day, by using one of the longer audio tools in this book or taking a short nap (we'll cover the art of napping in Week 5).

By thinking in cycles instead of hours, you are helping your brilliant circadian rhythm to stay on track. Sleep is so much more than just eight hours or else.

Sleep chapters

Sleep changes over time and varies according to circumstances. It changes from week to week, month to month and year to year. In fact, we experience fluctuating sleep health, or what I call sleep chapters, throughout our lives.

You have probably already experienced so many different kinds of sleep, from night to night, week to week. You may have had turbulent nights full of dreamy, other-worldly experiences; stressed and pressured sleep; and regular, simple, easy-but-adequate sleep. I'm sure that like most of us you've had short and fragmented nights when you were ill and when your immune system was mobilising its internal immunity to aid the recovery of your body.

You may find it reassuring to hear that no one has the same

Sleep changes throughout life

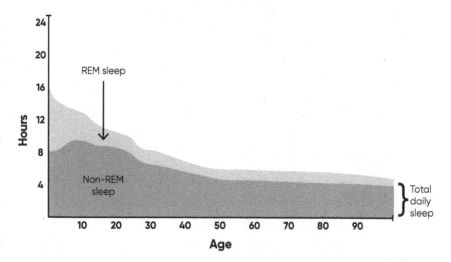

perfect sleep from birth to final resting place. Sleep struggles are universal. There's no right or wrong. We don't fix our sleep – or any other aspect of our health – at one perfect point throughout our lives. We need to learn to connect with it and understand our unique sleep health and what it means for us.

Pioneering sleep science studies back this up, showing that our sleep needs adapt and change over a lifetime.[5] While we can't control all these changes, we can help to ease any stress by supporting ourselves with how we respond. The image above depicts the general changes of sleep depth and duration across our lifespan.

We all fall somewhere on the bell-shaped curve of sleep need, depending on age, genetics and the context of your life. The Sleep Reset will help you to establish the right healthy, consistent sleep for you in each chapter of life.

Bhavin came to me seeking help to overcome spiralling sleep worries and episodes of what he believed to be work-related insomnia. A racing mind, agitated sleep and waking in the early hours were all regular occurrences. Bhavin told me he needed distractions in order to sleep and was worried his sleep health was getting worse.

We uncovered significant sleep chapters in Bhavin's past that proved to be huge red flags. He was diagnosed with myalgic encephalomyelitis (ME, aka chronic fatigue syndrome) at the age of seven, which led to increased parental soothing and a huge health emphasis on getting lots of sleep. A twin, he remembered being put to bed earlier than his brother and defining success as very long sleeps. Sleep for Bhavin was loaded with success and, when we explored his language, he realised that sleep was, and had been, a competition his entire life.

Remarkably, he grew out of ME, his energy levels improved and he was thriving in a busy career with high value and meaning to him, but this sleep stress hangover needed attention. Bhavin hadn't acknowledged that he had had great success with sleep even if it took a little longer sometimes for him to transition down into sleep. He had forgotten that there wasn't a medal to chase!

Taking the chance to understand his experiences of sleep in the past while adapting his thinking for the future removed the mental stress of sleep.

Accepting that we all have sleep challenges and different sleep chapters is at the very heart of a brand-new sleep health mindset, a pathway towards enhanced sleep health.

ACTION: **CHANGING YOUR SLEEP NARRATIVE**

Below are five steps to creating a more helpful sleep narrative. You can practise this comforting exercise at night before you go to bed, if you wake in the early hours and when you wake up. Just like any new skill, the more you practise, the more you embed your healthy relationship with sleep and hit 'refresh' on your sleep mindset.

- Step 1: Present: choose to bring visual focus to a single point in front of you or lower your gaze, resting your attention on just one thing while you settle into this moment.

- Step 2: Past: concentrate on imagining yourself in a past sleep struggle. Focus on a past point of sleep frustration and recognise your exhausted sleep anxiety . . . 'There is nothing I can do', 'I just can't sleep', etc.

- Step 3: Float: now imagine that you are floating to the side of yourself or watching yourself on a small screen moving away but with awareness. See if you can observe how unhelpful it is to burden yourself unnecessarily with pressure, sleep expectation and irritation.

- Step 4: Turn down the sound: imagine you could turn down the volume on your internal self-talk. Now fade this old, habitual sleep story in your mind and take slower, deeper breaths.

- Step 5: Update your sleep story: take six deep breaths while rehearsing a new sleep story in your mind – this might look like:

  - 'I can choose a positive Sleep Reset.'

  - 'I look forward to good sleep quality.'

  - 'I can learn to sleep deeply.'

  - 'I will focus on deeper sleep well-being.'

We know that our thinking styles and mindsets can actually help shape our health behaviours and become a positive influence on our sleep. Not only does changing your style of thinking help you in your conscious mind, it also creates neuroplasticity, which, in simple terms, is our brilliant brain's natural ability to change across our lifetime in response to our environment and thinking. This allows you to shift and orient your behaviour and thoughts more easily.

This is a subtle shift, but being aware can transform everything. Instead of labelling yourself a bad sleeper, think of your relationship with sleep as something to be understood, to be reset with connection and self-awareness.

HABITS CHANGE FASTER WITH A KIND MINDSET.

THE SLEEP STRESS THINKING TRAP

The way you think about your sleep and how you manage stress every day really matters. Let me unpack that for you. Before actions and habits, everything always starts with a belief and then a thought, and both can be changed for the better. Therefore, no matter how you are feeling about your sleep, you can always respond with ways to update your thinking and make better habit choices.

Self-talk really matters; indeed, how we talk to ourselves is just as important as our external environment.

When we put our head on the pillow, we engage in disaster rehearsal thinking, which in turn fuels the fake news that we are not enough. This feeling that sleep is impossible is 'all-or-nothing' thinking, which usually plays loudest at night.

What starts as a fleeting thought at 3.30am can turn into an absolute, a definite, and despite the fact that it hasn't even happened yet, it becomes a self-fulfilling prophecy. As you 'spiral down', you close off options to the point where you start feeling like there's no other choice available. It goes from a 'what if' to an 'I'm not' or 'I won't'.

'I'm terrible at sleeping, it's hopeless, I knew this was going
   to happen.'
'I can't sleep right now, I'm hot and my mind's whirring.'
'I won't sleep for hours, I can feel it.'
'I'll never sleep through this.'
'I'm stuck, here we go again.'
'Today will be terrible.'
'It's not going to be fixed.'
'Sleep's broken.'
'I'm stuck.'
'Alone.'
'Awake.'

Understanding your spiral down will help you to unpick what
sleeplessness is to you. This spiral of unhelpful thoughts takes you
further away from essential rest and recovery. You become your
own unhelpful mind coach, visualising bad performance, poor connection and having a really bad day.

Your fatigue voice

The fatigue voice is quite different from the voice you hear when
you're feeling at your most resilient. And when we pay attention to
this tired voice, it creates a cascade of unhealthy thinking and
coping strategies: more caffeine, more scrolling, more stress, more
distraction and more burnout.

Leo, a busy CEO, told me: 'I was sleeping for just two to three
hours a night, which affected my mood and my behaviour. I started to
have performance anxiety and to second-guess my skill and position.
Every thought made me feel like a zombie on autopilot. The effort of
coping was overwhelming. I felt tired but completely wired, unable to
sleep even when I had the opportunity. My mind kept predicting terrible consequences for my work performance.'

As a coach and therapist, every day I encourage people to learn
the skills to become aware of the unhelpful thinking traps and
habitual loops in their everyday behaviour. It's no coincidence we

see this more when experiencing insomnia, depression and anxiety. Sleep affects mood and mood affects sleep.

Every day, you probably verbalise or internalise your experience of being sleep-shattered in your own tired voice: 'I'm so tired', 'I'm exhausted', 'I feel burned out' or 'I'm completely knackered', together with accompanying sighs. But you are experiencing much more in your fatigued mind than simply being tired. Perhaps you feel unusually low, emotional, reactively up and down, constantly anxious or worried?

ACTION: IDENTIFY YOUR FATIGUE VOICE

- What is your fatigue voice?

- Does this become worse when you're experiencing sleep turbulence or limited sleep as a result of work-related stress or family problems?

- Do you notice or consider how you talk about sleep when things are going well – if you talk about sleep at all?

Continuous sub-quality sleep negatively shapes your focus and life, your body and mind, your work and relationships. You're living in a fog of poor well-being and, as a result, you're missing out on your sleep potential.

The emotional connection

How do you think with your extremely weary, tired brain? Do you react impulsively when you feel exhausted and underslept, especially towards those you love? In group sessions and one-to-ones, people tell me that, besides alertness, the thing they care about the most is how they are with the people in their life. How they show up for others bothers them a lot, as does the impact this has on their work and home life. There's often a feeling of shame and hopelessness. Even without insomnia, being poorly slept is a disadvantage in all aspects of health and well-being.

Amelia, a nurse, told me she didn't want to be explosive and reactive with her partner and teenage daughter. She wanted to show up for her colleagues and patients too. Sleepless, we feel far away from our natural patience and compassion and we seem to argue more. In Amelia's case, she cared less about the physical effects of being tired; it was sleep's effect on her behaviour and emotional well-being that was crushing her self-esteem, driving her to despair and ultimately fuelling her feeling of being stuck.

Research has shown that sleep deprivation leads to lower alertness and difficulties with daytime focus and concentration.[6] Underslept, we descend into emotional reactivity, making less useful choices, which can spiral into anxious thoughts, negativity and low mood.

Left unchecked, these thinking loops can mess up our sleep through hyperarousal (a state of high alert) and feeding what we call 'faulty' thinking, adding to further sleep distress.

One of the best ways to break this thinking trap is to harness the power of your breath, and box breathing is a really simple way to do this. You can start practising box breathing straightaway before moving on to the three-minute Calming Box Energy Reset tool on page 56.

BOX BREATHING

If you don't think you're 'good' at relaxing, try box breathing. This effortless technique taps into your natural relaxation response and is a gateway habit to realising you *can* slow down.

- Breathe in for four seconds.

- Hold your breath for four seconds.

- Exhale for four seconds.

- Pause for four seconds before taking your next breath.

REFRAMING YOUR SLEEP

It might be that you feel stuck because you've always been told you've got sleep problems and had an episode of five years on sleeping tablets. Even though, since then, you've had 15 years of sleeping well, your experience will always make you feel that sleep is hard for you. Or it could be that you've never really paid attention to sleep and have just been accepting that it's been all over the shop. You might even love a goal and a focus and want to know everything there is to know about sleep, follow my method verbatim and believe you can change quite quickly. None of these beliefs are wrong. In fact, very often, focusing on mindset and sleep is beneficial no matter what your sleep story.

We can opt to create a new mindset by leaving behind judgement or self-talk that is unfairly negative and creates sleep stress. This reframing of your sleep is helpful in switching focus from sleep 'loss', or what you think you have lost, to what you've gained, even if it is not the optimum amount of sleep *just yet*.

If you ignore your pain or hurt yourself with self-criticism, you're allowing your sleep and rest to be deprioritised. Instead, acknowledge that you will never have total control over whatever is going to disturb your sleep, but by simply noticing and being kind to yourself, you can stop the spiral. You have a choice over how you respond.

Just by having different thoughts and stopping judging yourself, you can influence your physiology and return to a more neutral state of mind.

NO MATTER HOW YOU ARE FEELING ABOUT YOUR SLEEP, YOU CAN ALWAYS CHANGE YOUR STYLE OF THINKING.

A great way to start exploring your own sleep mindset is through self-inquiry. Self-inquiry is the heart of evidence-based mindfulness programmes and is the practice of asking questions without judgement in the here and now, investigating your experience both in your thoughts and your body.

Much like the incredibly well-researched mindfulness-based interventions for anxiety and depression, seminal research around mindfulness and fMRI scans of the brain offer some helpful new approaches to lift you out of the sleep stress thinking trap.[7] Recent studies show that regular mindfulness practices can positively alter our brain in our resting state with lasting effects.[8]

This week's highly effective sleep audio tools (page 54) will help you train your mindset, feel empowered and guide you to rewind deep mind habits and limiting beliefs. Hypnosis visualisations move us forward into new spaces of possibility deep within our mind, beyond self-doubt, and update that inner soundtrack that's holding us back. The 'Releasing Stress from Sleep' audio tool (page 54) will allow you to open your mind to new potential and turn these 'spiral down' loops on their head.

Choosing to grow this positive mindset, and resetting your trust in yourself as a natural sleeper – for you are on your way to becoming one – will allow you to make the small changes in behaviour that will help you to achieve this.

Here's Leo again, talking about how changing his inner voice made a difference to him: 'The real revelation was learning ways to reframe the negative internal chatter that felt so loud in the middle of the night.'

Like Leo, you will also become your own sleep coach. Do you think a good sleep coach would judge their client? Or criticise them? You already have a kind and helpful mindset towards those you care about. Tuning into that mindset and offering it to yourself in times of need is an essential skill. How would you be with an exhausted child, a partner, friend or loved one? You'd likely tell them to lie down, have a nap, relax, have an early night, reschedule or take a breather. Extend that same kindness to yourself – you matter.

How to change unfriendly sleep thoughts

Let's take a look below at some examples of self-defeating thoughts I come across that can make sleep more pressured and fuel insomnia:

- 'I need exactly eight hours of unbroken sleep.'
- 'Insomnia is ruining my ability to enjoy life.'
- 'I cannot function after a night of bad sleep.'
- 'Insomnia will have serious health consequences.'
- 'One night of broken sleep will disrupt my entire week.'
- 'If I spend more time in bed, I will get more sleep.'
- 'I have lost control over my ability to sleep.'
- 'I need to cancel appointments or social engagements after a night of insomnia.'

If you have self-defeating thoughts like those above, perhaps you can you choose to recycle them and put them to better use. With a simple switch you can ease your mindset and aid insomnia recovery. Learning to recognise and change negative sleep thoughts through cognitive recycling simply means replacing unfriendly sleep thoughts with more helpful, moment-by-moment thoughts about sleep. Negative thoughts are usually distorted by stress and you can choose to disperse them by trying the exercise below, which I call 'catch it, cool it, choose it'. Let's start with the catastrophising, self-defeating thought: *If I don't get any sleep tonight, tomorrow I'll freeze in my presentation . . . I will be extremely anxious; I can't do this.*

- Catch it: 'I am just having a thought about the future; this is only my tired worry voice.'
- Cool it: 'I know tired. In the past I have handled poor sleep. I have a choice to rest now.'
- Choose it: 'I can always choose to rest regardless of my sleep tonight. In the morning, I can choose to get up and practise my Sleep Reset audio tools.'

These more accurate, positive beliefs will diffuse your sleep anxiety and reduce the worries that can trigger your sleep stress.

ACTION: RECYCLE SELF-DEFEATING THOUGHTS

Self-talk matters because it can take you into an unhelpful mindset around your sleep.

- Notice the language you use.

- Is it helpful or can you see there is space to change, reflect and connect?

- Can you use the 'catch it, cool it, choose it' method to recycle your negative thoughts?

'OUR MINDS AREN'T PASSIVE OBSERVERS SIMPLY OBSERVING REALITY AS IT IS; OUR MINDS ACTUALLY CHANGE REALITY. THE REALITY WE EXPERIENCE TOMORROW IS PARTLY THE PRODUCT OF THE MINDSETS WE HOLD TODAY.'

DR ALIA CRUM, ASSOCIATE PROFESSOR OF PSYCHOLOGY AT STANFORD UNIVERSITY AND DIRECTOR OF THE STANFORD MIND & BODY LAB[9]

I hope you are starting to grasp that there is no pass or fail here, only a journey or transition towards strengthening your sleep. As I stressed earlier, instead of rushing into change, let's reflect in order to build a meaningful mindset that will work for you.

In Week 2, we'll discover the science behind sleep and how important the cycle of light and dark is to our biological clock and the sleep–wake cycle.

WEEK 1 SLEEP RESET TOOLKIT

Meet this week's Sleep Reset tools, designed to help you absorb this chapter and set the scene to change your relationship with sleep for the better, building that strong foundation to personal sleep health – your sleeping mindset.

YOUR WEEK 1 TOOLKIT RECOVERY MENU

- Your Mindset Tool: The Deep Sleep Body Scan (5-minute guided audio download)

- Your Breathing Tool: The Calming Box Energy Reset (3-minute guided audio download)

- Your Sleep Hypnosis: Releasing Stress from Sleep (7-minute guided audio download)

These are all easy wins as everything is guided and recorded for you to layer into action.

These tools will help you do five things really well:

1. Reframe your relationship to sleep (your mindset).
2. Begin to reignite your natural deep recovery skills as you become more aware of change starting to take place.
3. Help you feel empowered.
4. Enable you to sleep deeper.
5. Teach you that habit-changing kryptonite – self-kindness.

You may notice that the tools this week encourage you to wind down. Relaxation is naturally a given – but it is not the only goal. Ultimately, these tools will work on a deep level to help build back your trust in sleep and help you focus on your sleep health. They help put this whole chapter into action for you – by practising the tools you are already taking committed action to strengthen your sleeping mindset.

Your Mindset Tool: The Deep Sleep Body Scan

Developing a consistent way to begin resting your body on command is a key building block for your Sleep Reset. This is your foundational recovery tool and an essential first step in your sleep well-being toolkit.

The main intention of this body scan is to learn to centre your mind and thoughts down into a body-and-breath sensory experience. In this exercise, you will practise a multi-layered technique that starts with some connected breathing and then allows you to deepen your focus with a sleep scan infused with deep sleep suggestion, helping you direct the relaxation response.

The Deep Sleep Body Scan is a mind and body technique of starting relaxation from the feet first to help dial down your busy thinking and planning mind. This is a dynamic relaxation tool that helps with guiding your attention and focus and is an easy win to get on board with if you frequently feel tired but wired. Your pre-sleep bedtime is therefore the perfect training ground to practise this.

Do this exercise with purpose, ideally in the late evening as a five-minute wind-down strategy towards sleep. However, there is never a wrong time to tune into your body, so feel free to do this scan at any time of the day.

Ideally do this as a lying-down practice this week as you learn to just be still momentarily and at peace with yourself.

Over and over, the research shows that having a mind–body tool that helps you relate to your physical body is amazing for both stress reduction and managing recurring anxiety and depression, and is something we very often overlook in our everyday lives, especially at night.[10]

Here you'll practise your version of settling into recovery mode: stillness. In neuroscience, a body scan is usefully often referred to as 'non-sleep deep rest', or NSDR, a term coined by academic Dr Andrew Huberman.[11] This highlights the powerful effects that we can create when we practise this type of science-based recovery tool.

Be patient with your attention as you scan – you've got this.

> This is the first of many body scans in the book. Each has a unique tweak depending on the theme of the week, but the focus this week is on building that strong mind-body relaxation response.

This tool is brilliant for:

- calming a racing mind
- training your mind–body–breath muscle
- helping you disconnect from a busy mind
- reconnecting with your body and getting used to being still and relaxed in your bed
- easing tension and anxiety

You can layer this up the following morning with a super-effective entry point into connected breathwork – the three-minute Calming Box Energy Reset. I find clients like this clear, easy-to-follow tool as it's very simple to adopt.

Your Breathing Tool: The Calming Box Energy Reset

Welcome to your first breathing check-in – an everyday way for you to energise after sleep, wake up, reset and set the tone for the day. This exercise is an easy entry point into harnessing the power of the breath to support your sleep. The perfect time to do this is as soon as you get up and open the curtains.

This tool helps you build some intention into your waking day instead of reaching for your phone as soon as you wake up and reacquaints you with box breathing (see page 49), or perhaps helps you refresh your breathing habits that are helpful for sleep.

Top tip: you can also use this box breathing exercise to respond to fleeting sleeplessness or wake-ups.

Through this practical breathing exercise, I guide you step by step. Just allow yourself the gift of a little patience, space and time as I guide you into observing your breath and your posture as you find it. This can become a moment-by-moment check-in and is a really helpful way to step out of a busy mind and back into a calmer and more grounded body through breathing awareness.

The exhale holds the real power, sending a signal to our brain and body that we are not under threat and encouraging us to develop a more useful recovery response, providing respite from imagined stressors or our current reality. In this way, we can find more choice in how to respond and create a secure breathing space, a place of safety away from danger, to anchor back down into.

You can practise relaxing and guiding your breath in more helpful ways during the day. Reset and spend just one moment noticing your posture and state of mind. Find the space where you feel a little calmer, much clearer and quite different from three minutes before.

ACTION: **PLAN FOR SLEEP RESET SUCCESS**

What current morning habit can you 'coat hanger' this breathwork onto so it becomes a 'sleep well tonight' habit? For example, as an energising wake-up ritual, post-teeth clean, when you make your morning cuppa or every time you shut your front door.

Write your intention below:

'I will realistically and deliberately do this every time I
_____ or when I _____'

SEE THE MIND-BODY THOUGHT LOOP AT PLAY

In recognition that these evidence-based mind-body tools – otherwise known as hypnosis, meditation and visualisation – may be brand new to you, or something you've heard of but put in the 'sceptical' box in your mind, let me help break it down for you. Most people have the ability to visualise – to call up on command – a cinematic image of a prompt. You can do this right now. If I asked you to recall the following questions, you would have to use your imagination and visualisation to answer them:

- Do you like the colour of your front door?

- What side is the keyhole?

- Do you like eating lemons? (Nearly everyone adds in a facial motion when answering this one!)

Most people can do this – you already have these inbuilt skills; I am asking you to put them to use for your sleep health. This is an example of the mind-body loop in action.

Hypnosis is superb at helping us bypass the self-critical judging mind and it's the most effective way to reframe situations and challenges, propelling us forward into spaces of new potential in our mind. By focusing on what we are 'for' rather than what we are 'against' – in other words, concentrating on our health goals and what we can change rather than staying stuck in our autopilot habits – hypnosis can help us create a positive path forward. This is less about falling asleep at the moment of hypnosis and more about changing our negative thoughts about sleep so that, when night-time arrives, we're able to nod off without issue.

Your Sleep Hypnosis: Releasing Stress from Sleep

This tool can help to improve several measures of psychological well-being whether it is practised in the morning or evening.

This is the first hypnotherapy experience of the Sleep Reset and is about finding space in your mind for recovery and to create a sleep well-being approach for yourself.

The skill practised in this sleep hypnotherapy is learning to sit down with a recurring stressful feeling that is holding you back from sleep and learning how to respond and not react with stress.

Working on these essential skills is a little like this:

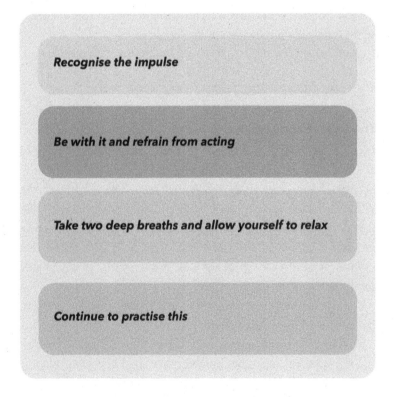

Recognise the impulse

Be with it and refrain from acting

Take two deep breaths and allow yourself to relax

Continue to practise this

Noticing you are tired means you can choose to rest for a minute and reset your breathing. Slowing down your breathing will help your nervous system.

Make a commitment to yourself and choose two nights to bring this tool into your bedtime ritual. This tool alone will be highly beneficial and means you'll take a giant leap forward in learning to relax. It's useful to remember that we don't stress ourselves to sleep; we relax ourselves to sleep – and this is why hypnosis is superb as it helps you build up your relaxation skills. It's a skill you can return to time and again to relax your mind and body.

There's no right or wrong way here. You may want to do this an hour before bedtime or just as your head hits the pillow. Equally, if you want to do this every night this week, feel free, but starting small helps you to take action. Simply make the choice that's right for you. Put it in your diary or set an alarm to remind you. The transcript is hosted on www.mindtonicsleep.com.

YOUR WEEK 1 BONUS TOOLS

The Reset fist pump

It's great to know from the start that positive reinforcement really helps over shame and judgement when it comes to making healthy changes. Study after study shows that self-celebration beats the self-critic hands down for well-being and deep habit change – this is also true for your sleep health.[12] In fact, listening to the self-critic mindset is correlated with increased stress, poor self-control, less motivation and poor self-belief – all really unhelpful ingredients for improving your sleep.[13]

This is so important for you to acknowledge when changing habits or working on your goals.

With that in mind, how do you typically celebrate your success during the precious but humble everyday? I bet that made you think. We easily know how we celebrate the traditions, holidays, the big stuff, but what about those little everyday wins? I know you stress and sweat the small stuff, so what's the opposite?

Fast forward time for a moment to celebrating your Sleep Reset achievements. What do you look like? How will you know? It's good to imagine the possibility and upside of the next few weeks.

Imagine if you had a new way to celebrate the end of your day and the arrival of your recovery time. How would that transform the purpose of your time, away from autopilot late-night tech habits? This concept always gets my clients really reimagining the humble weeknight. How could you celebrate the end of the day with some meaning? This could look like simple things such as lighting a candle, writing in your journal or harnessing the benefits of an evening stroll (which you'll learn more about in Week 2).

Do not shy away from doing this – I encourage you to be deliberate in this often overlooked recovery tool.

If you start the day fully committed and end it fully committed (not to me but to yourself – to your sleep health), I want you to celebrate your success. It's also a really great way to keep accountable and come back to your sleep story and Sleep Reset at times of need.

This is the self-compassion element in action – you are never alone.

Instant mind boost

We've established that you already have a PhD in your own unique (usually negative) self-talk. I want to share one of the most profound tools to help you reset your self-talk. If you're really struggling with sleep and a judgemental mindset, this effortless bonus tool can accelerate your positive self-belief and facilitate self-awareness and self-kindness – that one habit that I know you don't practise enough.

It takes just ten mindset-priming seconds in the morning and at bedtime.

Repeat after me: 'I like myself.'
'I like myself when I do . . .'
'I really like myself when I cope with . . .'

Go further: 'I like my whole self.'
'I love myself.'
'I accept myself and all my imperfections.'

Top tip: saying it aloud is impossible to do through gritted teeth!

Practise this anytime, especially when alone:

- every wake-up before you pick up your phone
- every time you put down your phone
- every time your head touches the pillow

When it comes to habit change, self-kindness is key.

YOUR REALISTIC SLEEP RESET 'PRESCRIPTION'

If you're super tired and would like me to prescribe the best strong start to your Reset, here is what your week might look like:

Tool	Monday	Tuesday	Wednesday	Thursday	Friday	Saturday (optional)	Sunday
Mindset	✓ (morning)	✓		✓ (morning)	✓ (morning)		✓
Breathing	✓ (mid-afternoon)		✓	✓ (mid-afternoon)	✓ (morning)		✓
Sleep Hypnosis	✓ (bedtime)			✓ (bedtime)		✓	✓

I suggest you work with what's realistic for you and your best energy. Choose the days when you have the least friction (for example, if you know your weekends are busy, steer away from them). Start with small wins. If you can manage all three tools on two days and a Sunday or Monday sleep hypnosis, this will set your sleep mindset in motion.

Tear out, photocopy or take a photo of this page so you have a good overview of what the next seven days could look like.

WEEK 2: HARNESSING CIRCADIAN SCIENCE

In Week 1 you did invaluable work looking at your past and current sleep story. You've gained a new perspective and, crucially, a clearer focus on how to break out of sleep struggles by cutting loose the self-defeating thoughts you've had about sleep that have been holding you back.

This week we will focus on understanding your circadian rhythm (your body clock), the impact of light and darkness and choosing a sleep-friendly approach to day and night.

YOU ARE ALREADY THE OWNER OF THE MOST EVOLVED SLEEP TECH ON EARTH: YOUR INNER BODY CLOCK. LET'S PUT IT TO GOOD USE.

GETTING TO KNOW YOUR INTERNAL 'SLEEP TECH'

You have two independent but beautifully fluent sleep processes working together for you, not against you, always seeking to deliver beneficial sleep (even if right now it doesn't feel like enough). This is known as the two-part process – C and S – originally proposed in 1982 by the Swiss sleep researcher A.A. Borbély, and it provides a simple way for us to understand how sleep is generated and maintained across the night.[1]

Process C: your circadian rhythm

In a nutshell, circadian rhythms are physical, mental and behavioural changes that follow a 24-hour cycle. These natural processes respond primarily to light and dark and affect animals, plants and microbes too. From the moment you wake up, your body clock is sensing environmental light and dark cues as well as more subtle cues from food, temperature and even the timing of exercise (we'll cover this in Weeks 3 and 5). So evolved is this inner sleep tech that, through specialised sensors in the back of our eyes (intrinsically photosensitive retinal ganglion cells, or ipRGCs), it's also sensing where we are in the seasons.

Process C influences and synchs up the suprachiasmatic nucleus master clock, located deep within a tiny region of your brain's hypothalamus, which is the central pacemaker of the circadian timing system. This is your principal circadian clock, directing the daily cycles of behaviour and physiology that set the tempo of your life.[2] I call this master clock our very own tiny 'Big Ben'. Process C can be reset by timing our exposure to light and dark (more on this later).

Often, the notion of our circadian rhythm is part of our common knowledge, but the vast majority of my clients are unsure of how to make sleep science work for them. In my experience, when clients familiarise themselves with circadian science it really helps to get them motivated about their sleep health potential.

I find it impactful to explain circadian rhythms as your very own invisible code for performance. This internal timekeeping supports your day and night, guiding daily physical, brain, body and behavioural processes, and is a vital guiding force for our sleep system.[3]

Most living creatures possess this highly intelligent circadian timing system. Important new insights continue to show that circadian rhythms are everywhere in our biology, and a study in 2021 even found circadian clocks in our heart cells, which help to change heart function across its own 24-hour circadian cycle.[4]

Biologically hardwired in, circadian rhythms help us thrive and adapt to shifting seasons and the environment we live in. They help our brain and body cycle through day and night, thriving on light timing and exposure, something we seem to have long forgotten to pay attention to in the fast-paced, brightly lit 24/7 digital ocean that is our modern world.

Simply put, light governs our entire internal biology – even the microbiome in our gut has its own clock – and, finally, we are beginning to understand that circadian health impacts sleep pathways in stunning ways.[5]

This circadian timing system timetables all our important functions such as cognition capabilities, mood, energy, focus and immune function, hormone releasing, digestion and eating habits and, critically for our sleep system, core body temperature (more on this on page 65).

Process S: sleep pressure

The second process is sleep pressure. From the moment we wake up, we start producing a chemical called adenosine, which gradually builds up and creates a natural sleep pressure. I like to think of it as a timer or weighted blanket that helps you feel sleepy, generally 16–18 hours after waking up.

As sundown occurs, we start producing melatonin, a hormone primarily released at night by the pineal gland in the brain, which influences the rhythm of our sleep–wake cycle, allowing us to experience good-quality sleep. Our master clock (tiny Big Ben) controls how much melatonin is produced based on light levels detected by the retinas in our eyes. Melatonin production generally peaks from mid-evening onwards before decreasing in the early hours of the morning. Before we actually wake up, we are already building cortisol, which will bring us out of sleep into being wide awake (more on this later too).

You can consider melatonin actually functioning like a clock hand on our master clock, keeping us to a regular sleep–wake cycle. In simple terms, it provides an early 'let's head into night mode' cue.

This is why the longer we're awake, the more natural pressure there is to fall asleep. This continuous cycle between S and C means that, when we fall asleep again, the pressure is relieved and the cycle of sleep–wake–sleep–repeat continues when our sleep health is in good shape.[6]

While melatonin levels are greatest at night, it is still present in tiny amounts during the daytime. It is localised within our mitochondria – the energy powerhouse of our cells – acting as a powerful antioxidant during the day.

THE GENDER DIFFERENCE

It may surprise you to hear that sleep research has shown a subtle difference in the circadian timing system between different genders. The average circadian rhythms of melatonin and core body temperature are set to an earlier hour in women than in men, even when both sexes maintain almost identical and consistent bedtimes and wake-up times.[7]

Women especially report suffering negative effects when their circadian rhythm is interrupted. They tend to wake up earlier than men and exhibit a greater preference for morning activities than men. In my clinic, I often see the impact of undiagnosed sleep issues in women.

Process S: sleep pressure is why you find the longer you're awake, the more you will feel an inner urge or sleep pressure signal urging you to sleep. From the moment you wake up in the morning, it helps you build a sleep appetite as sleep pressure gradually builds up during the day and sharply drops as soon as we fall asleep, ready to repeat again in the morning.

Process C: circadian sleep timing is managed by our internal, tiny Big Ben body clock. Process C provides an overall timing mechanism for our sleep regulation linked to our exposure to Earth's 24-hour rotation cycle.

Our circadian rhythm or internal body clock's main mission is to help us thrive and predict behaviours needed for survival and well-being. Our body clock is hardwired by evolution and coded to track the sun and seasons. The circadian rhythm is more precious than any other alarm and it also tells all our cells the perfect time to be in action or what to do.

If we can keep a regular biological night and day schedule – so a 'normal' sleep–wake routine – this tag team works in blissful harmony, but sometimes the two processes can decouple, creating sleep challenges and a well-being nightmare. (An obvious example you may already have experienced when Processes C and S are out of alignment is jet lag.)

Our circadian system doesn't just help balance our 24-hour sleep–wake cycle, it impacts all internal health deep down to cellular level, influencing our immune function, metabolism, hormone and reproduction systems, heart rate, blood sugar and pressure, cognition and mood.

The reality of life in our permanently switched-on world means we need to learn, relearn or be reminded of the basics behind our sleep physiology and the non-negotiable importance of sleep. Learning more about our body clocks reminds us just how intimately we are connected with natural day–night cycles.

It's essential we learn to work in harmony and ease with these inner sleep tech systems and not against them, for there is no escaping the health challenges we will face if we continue to live long term with a poor light environment and debilitated sleep health.[8]

Light's ability to reset and swing the body clock

Every day, light influences our circadian biology. Light in the morning helps stabilise and reset your body clock and other circadian rhythms, while bright light later at night will subtly delay your body clock and sleep. Daytime sunlight is vital for every aspect of our health and our sleep–wake cycle, impacting nearly every organ of our body, from our skin and hair to our liver and intestines. This is why the right timing and exposure of light and dark is so vital for sleep well-being, impacting our sleep quality, timing and duration of our overnight sleep as well as our wider circadian health.[9]

NATURE'S OWN SLEEP AID

Bluer light in the morning - like a morning sky - gives a boost of energy and helps you to get out of bed.

Daytime light, or bright light, with cooler tones helps signal to your body that it's time to be alert and helps with productivity.

Then at the end of the day, the amber colours of a sunset help prepare you for sleep and signal melatonin to rise.[10]

Excuse me for a moment while I geek out on the sleep science. Circadian rhythm and light expert Dr Samer Hattar coined the phrase: 'Take a photon instead of a pill.'[11] While studying the inner retina in mammals' eyes, he and his team discovered how viewing light at particular times directly influences much more than just being awake or asleep. They were pivotal in investigating a subset of light-sensitive specialist eye cells (or ipRGCs) that help synch up our circadian rhythms with the outside world.[12]

The visual below shows that, from the moment you wake, you're building your sleep potential:

Sleep/Wake Regulation

Even before we wake up, our inner sleep tech is already monitoring and sensing light, informing the brain to taper off melatonin production. Our body then begins to warm and starts producing cortisol and adrenaline. This takes us into the transition from sleep to wake mode known as the 'cortisol awakening response' (CAR) effect, whereby our brain and body release our biggest timed dose of natural cortisol. This cortisol pulse effect lasts for around 30 minutes before we feel fully awake.[13]

We need this huge shower of healthy cortisol to be released into the blood system and up into areas of the brain to increase energy. We cannot override this: each and every one of us has this invisible morning shower coded in and these high levels of cortisol are written into our genome. This process is crucial, helping to balance our powerful circadian rhythm and our body clock system (Process C, page 65) in harmony with sleep pressure (Process S, page 66).

We often misjudge cortisol as purely a stress hormone, which isn't the full picture. I encourage my clients to think of cortisol as a hormone of energy. As scientific research shows, it produces an alerting signal whereby even if we don't immediately feel like eating, we want to move to find food. It also signals an increased breathing and heart rate.[14]

Cortisol and adrenaline are also powerful regulators of energy, helping us maintain good immune system function. Morning cortisol is the waking agent we need to help us focus alongside healthy dopamine and many other neurotransmitters, which ease us into our day and encourage healthy sleep at night.

HARNESSING THE POWER OF LIGHT

We are biologically a diurnal species – coded to be daylight active and naturally sleep and restore with darkness overnight. The problem I often see is that we just aren't getting enough of the right light at the correct times for sleep well-being, subconsciously dysregulating ourselves from our inner sleep tech.

In many global studies, it appears that our society is evolving to be an indoor species, shielded from the supportive effects of natural light and sunlight.[15] While a typical classroom, office or hospital setting provides a light intensity that is between 150 and 1,000 lux (a measurement of light intensity), being outside on a sunny day can mean being exposed to light that is 10 to 1,000 times brighter. The variation in brightness between indoor and outdoor environments is not always obvious because our eyes are very good at adjusting to different light levels.

Indoor lighting in our homes and workplaces really has a powerful impact in both helpful and hindering ways. We spend on average over 90 per cent of our days indoors in the Western world.[16] It feels quite shocking when you think about it, and I know that stat stays in my mind as a helpful nudge to take work calls or mind breaks outside or near a window as often as possible.

Now ask yourself whether your busy, always-on life is creating a confusing 'lightmare' for your circadian system and perhaps throwing off your sleep potential. If your internal body clock gets thrown off from working in a windowless office or from jet lag, it's only a matter of time before your sleep well-being and sleep at night start to suffer as a result of not receiving the environmental cues needed to produce good-quality sleep.

A good night's sleep starts the moment you wake up

I want you to shift your focus from falling asleep to waking up. I know it seems like a bit of a paradox, but your potential for better sleep starts the moment you wake up. Morning sunlight is the most powerful reset for our circadian health. Exposure to natural blue light – which helps the body wake up and is most potent in the morning – and daily sunlight across the morning is critical to regulating our circadian rhythms and training our clocks to keep a regular 24-hour biological 'beat'.

EACH MORNING CAN HELPFULLY BUILD A NEW NIGHT.

I have found that acknowledging this simple fact helps take the pressure off judging the sleep we've had the night before.

Light is the most important mechanism to synch our internal body clock to the outside world. As the days get longer in spring, for example, the light-sensitive ipRGC cells in our eyes detect and respond to this change. Waking to sunlight is more effective than getting up in darkness or snoozing in a bedroom with the curtains still shut or the blinds down. This is why we need the morning light sooner than most people realise – not just mid-morning, but ideally as soon as possible upon waking.

So powerful is the effect of light that a 2019 study found that exposure to morning sunlight results in greater alertness during the day, helping us to improve our health habits as well as leading to better sleep quality.[17] It also helps 'shake off' any feelings of sleep inertia – that natural sleep grogginess – while we experience our natural cortisol peak (that is like a natural caffeine boost). This initial dose of light tells the brain to shut down your overnight melatonin production and triggers the first dopamine release of the day. Your skin absorbs that natural sunlight and produces vitamin D, which helps nudge the production of dopamine as well as serotonin, meaning time in the sun can boost your dopamine levels and make you feel good on top of helping your sleep well-being. Producing these substances upon waking helps us feel naturally alert and allows cortisol and brain feel-good neurotransmitters, such as dopamine, norepinephrine and histamine, to rise.

Dr Samer Hattar's work and other recent research shows that our subconscious vision cells, or ipRGCs, also connect to the thalamus, an area of the brain related to mood.[18] With the pathways for sleep and mood overlapping by 90 per cent, it's not difficult to see why seeking natural morning light as a sleep health anchor much earlier in our daytime routine has positive benefits for our mind, body and mental health, from lowering blood pressure to improving our focus and regulating mood.[19]

Natural dawn light is the most powerful, but any outside light will have an outsized effect on your sleep in the night to come.[20] It comes as no surprise to me that a study showed that dog walkers enjoy regular good sleep, very possibly due to getting out in the natural sunlight early every morning.[21]

I would argue that seeking morning light is just as important as cleaning your teeth (and it's definitely more important for health than the detrimental daily habit of checking your phone!). It is one of the best free things that will help reset your sleep at night and prime your alertness during the day.

We can translate this research into easy-to-do actions. Think about the moment you wake up: could you open the curtains or raise the blinds within five minutes of waking? Could you have your cup of tea by the back door rather than in bed or in the kitchen? This is something that's really helped my sleep and means I can still access the beneficial effects of morning light, even on a cloudy day. Remember, our eyes need to view light and being outside will always be more effective than being inside by a window. These new morning habits alone have transformed the sleep of so many people I work with. It also feels really good, knowing that you're already improving your sleep chances later on at night.

Optimum exposure looks like 10–20 minutes on a clear day as soon as possible on waking – and, when it's cloudy, we should aim to be outside a little longer across the morning. Even on a grey, cloudy day, the light outside is hundreds of times more powerful than the light from a screen or the light indoors![22] If you can achieve 45–90 minutes on a cloudy day, it will be incredibly beneficial for your sleep well-being. Trying to build this into your morning is always preferable – that's what the science speaks to – but, more realistically, this could look like a morning walk if you don't have a commute, a couple of outside mini-breaks during the day and prioritising a lunch break outside. Remember, if you only do one or two of these things, you're already supporting your sleep tonight. Even two minutes outside begins to prime your body clocks in helpful ways, setting you on the right course for good sleep to come.

ACTION: NOURISH YOURSELF AT BREAKFAST WITH A HEALTHY DOSE OF DAYLIGHT

Think about HOW you can add to your morning light 'diet'. You can start promoting and supporting great sleep from the get-go by gifting yourself light as the ultimate healthy breakfast (along with a nutritious meal, of course)!

Start by seeking natural outside sunlight for a minimum of two to ten minutes every morning upon waking as often as you can, even on an overcast day. You can't beat heading outside first thing, but if you can't get outside, try to orient your workspace towards a window. If you can't, don't worry – as you'll come to learn, an evening walk will also help to keep your circadian rhythms on track (see page 105).

The easiest way to build this new morning light habit is to add it on to something that you habitually already do. The examples below will harness the inbuilt superpowers of your 'sleep well-being tech' as a proactive alternative to looking at your phone screen or hitting snooze!

- Every day, view the morning light as soon as possible after waking. Get up and open the blinds or curtains to help you feel alert faster, no matter what kind of sleep you had the night before. It takes just five seconds to boost your morning light consumption. Count back from five, taking big full breaths.

- In autumn and winter, use a bright light at home or a SAD lamp if you can (see pages 76–77).

- Seek the light before your brush your teeth.

- Enjoy a quick cuppa outside your front/back door (you don't need to go out in public). Ideally, take in the morning light without wearing sunglasses.

- Eat your breakfast as close as possible to some daylight or orient yourself towards the sky/light.

- Take a brisk early-morning walk around the block.

- Action some morning movement (exercise) outside through the seasons.

- Reset your morning commute to incorporate some daylight. For example, add in a five-minute walk or get off the bus one stop earlier.

Consistently choose to practise these easy morning steps. Priming your body clock outside will help to improve the quality and duration of your sleep, as well as your focus, performance, attention and learning ability. Morning light also acts as that all-important clock timer and prompt for the production of evening sleep melatonin.

Your potential for good sleep starts in the moment, not in the past. Right now, you can work with, not against, the life and health you deserve.

CONSIDER EACH TIME YOU WAKE UP AS AN OPPORTUNITY TO MAKE SUPPORTIVE HABIT AND BEHAVIOUR CHANGES IN LINE WITH YOUR CIRCADIAN BIOLOGY.[23]

Seeking light in the darker months

If it is autumn/winter and is still dark outside, morning light is even more essential to help us boost natural feel-good hormones and prompt our body clocks to be alert and energised.

When natural morning light is harder to come by, we can and must turn to our everyday home lights or lamps. Bright lightbulbs, especially overhead, are always naturally alerting or, if you can afford one, a sleep well-being light will simulate the sunlight-alerting effects when it is still dark outside. In the winter months, I use a sleep well-being light first thing. It is a desktop device that plugs in to illuminate my workspace, help prime good energy and attentive-ness and support my sleep–wake cycle. A cheaper way to do this is to use a ring 'selfie'-type light, easily found at a low cost online (generally only the price of two takeaway coffees and it will give you a much better boost!). This will have the same alerting effects until you can get outside for a natural mid-morning light break (see Resources, page 265.)

SAD LAMPS

One of the most well-known conditions whereby darker months impact our mental health and mood is seasonal affective disorder (SAD), which can cause low energy, listlessness and lethargy as well as deeper effects that really do feel like a seasonal depression (the winter blues). It is prevalent in approximately 5 per cent of the global population and, once again, we find there's a gender difference.[24] Researchers at the University of Glasgow found that women are much more likely than men to experience seasonal variations in depressive symptoms, with these peaking during the winter months.[25]

SAD lamps are specially designed tools that give a therapeutic dose of bright light. It's thought that when bright light hits the retina in the eye, the brain receives a message to reduce the pro-duction of melatonin. This can improve energy and mood. You need to orient yourself near one for at least 30 minutes each day to improve mood alertness and help anchor in your circadian rhythm. SAD lamps are around ten times the intensity of a normal domestic light. I use my portable light most of the year, moving it around the house and doing my morning exercise oriented towards this sleep health light. For me, it is like a portable sunshine boost that I can move around my work and living space during the daytime.

Bright light therapy is science-backed and is a sleep intervention in its own right in behavioural sleep medicine.[26] I would love to see artificial lighting that can replicate the biological effects of natural daylight within every workplace and home. This is the future of sleep health and it's brilliant that there are already some low-cost light therapy devices for our homes to help us in the darker seasonal months (see Resources, page 269).

Don't despair if getting outside first thing in the morning is hard. You still have the whole morning to seek some light where you can. I cannot emphasise just how important this is for your Sleep Reset and to help you absorb vitamin D – the sunshine vitamin that also supports your sleep system (see page 119).

THE WEEKEND SNOOZE REIMAGINED

Of course, just because you wake up and seek the light naturally doesn't mean that on the weekends you can't get back into your sleep space for breakfast in bed or to read a book. Many of my sleep clients and athletes love this time to practise some self-care with mind coaching and/or morning visualisations.

GUIDING EVENING LIGHT FOR BETTER SLEEP

Many of us further confuse our body clocks through the nature of our light 'diet' well into the evening. As the day progresses towards bedtime, the amount of light you get is within your control, especially last thing at night. The most unhelpful sources of light in the evening are blue light from electronic devices, which are proven to confuse and delay our sleep and keep the brain alert, and brightly lit bathrooms and bedrooms.[27]

Keep your bedroom low-tech

There is no doubt that our modern evenings are saturated with technology. You've seen that when people use their electronic devices in a dark environment, they are covered in a blue glow. That's high-energy visible light, and it's ready to disrupt everyone's sleep. While eye fatigue and sleep trouble may be the most commonly experienced problems associated with exposure to blue light, blue light late at night actually triggers a suppression of melatonin that is thought to impact learning and memory, disrupt our blood sugar regulation and even affect our gut–brain axis.[28]

I would encourage you to keep work and screens away from the bedroom and sleep time as best you can (and use a blue light blocker if you must – see page 268). Allowing brain-alerting news cycles, phone calls, texts and emails into our sleeping space is one of the worst things we can do and may act as a wake-up cue to our brains.

Aside from the light emitted, which acts as a handbrake to the sleepy feeling caused by our melatonin rising, blue-light technology creates a spike in our cortisol levels (see page 77) and also leads our brains to create a negative association with our bedroom, which subconsciously makes it more difficult to sleep there.

Spending hours late at night on mobile phones, tablets and computer screens consuming alerting blue-light technology soaks our evenings in sleep-blocking behaviours that subconsciously put the handbrake on sleep quality.

The research shows that blue light emitted by electronic devices suppresses the secretion of melatonin to some degree, but the worst time for this sleep-disrupting effect is between the later hours of 10pm and 4am, as a general guide.[29]

As the American neuroscientist Dr Andrew Huberman said: 'Avoid checking your phone in the middle of the night. The eye and brain clocks are very sensitive at night and the light signals to the body that it's still daytime, which can alter your sleep for several days. It's like jet lag: "If you're looking at your phone at 1am, you might as well have flown to Abu Dhabi."'[30]

Knowing that the effects of blue light on sleep quality can impact other elements of health and well-being is exactly the kind of insight that helps people keep their phone out of sight or away in a corner of the bedroom to stop that 1am or 4am sneak-peek scroll.

Choose a protective hour before bed

Having said all this, I am in no way anti-screens – and there is a good reason for this. I appreciate that we all need different ways to relax. Especially for my family, where we are neurodiverse and have teens, a total screen ban three hours before bed is not always helpful and actually creates tension at times.

Instead, we all agree to have an hour pre-sleep window – a non-negotiable time cutoff where we listen to music, read or take a long shower or deep bath to wind down in a way that is unique to us. It's doable, it's realistic and it's effective because we can all stick to it without any tension. There is no doubt in my mind that having a realistic approach that also has a clear boundary creates a huge uplift in self-care habits, connections and, in turn, better sleep quality.

What might this protective hour look like to you? Maybe you can wind down by scenting your home or sleep space with natural essential oils, investing in a deep rest with hypnotherapy, allowing more time for eye contact and screen-free connections, listening to music or an audiobook, or getting into bed with a good book. Reading a physical book before bed has consistently been shown to be incredible for sleep and general feelings of well-being and is an excellent way to relax the brain and fall asleep – studies show that reading can cut stress levels in half in about six minutes.[31] I find this really reassuring as it inspires me to pick up a book at bedtime, which means I'm less likely to see work emails or be tempted by online content. It's worth noting that using an e-reader, if that's your preference, is still better than scrolling on a much smaller phone device, particularly for eye strain.

My client Roz works at a tech start-up and had fallen into the classic 'wired but tired' trap. I'll let her describe her day in her own words:

'I'm great at early mornings and being go go go. I'm high energy throughout the day but, as soon as my head hits the pillow, I feel "razzed up" as I call it – my mind is charged and wired yet my body is tired and ready for sleep. I distract my mind by going back into work stuff on my phone, catching up with friends, scrolling and looking at social media. Then as I start to wind down, my partner wants to talk about big ticket stuff. It's all too much as I then go into planning mode, becoming even more wired and getting annoyed because I'm trying so hard to relax my busy mind.

'It takes me hours to fall asleep and, usually, I end up getting around five hours a night. I worry that this isn't sustainable long term. I'm living on adrenaline but don't tell me that tech is bad. I love tech – it's my life.'

I sensed instantly that I needed to help Roz rethink her bedtime routine. I showed her the connections with her internal tech, how our eyes process light and dark and how this influences our mind and body clock. Instead of strict sleep hygiene rules, I reminded her that she had a choice over her bedtime routine. My low-light tech guidance advised her to do any late-night work out of bed and in a chair instead, in a dimly lit bedroom wearing glasses designed to filter out the harmful blue-violet rays commonly emitted from digital screens (see Resources, page 268). She chose to continue scrolling through her non-work-related tech at bedtime as part of winding down but agreed with her partner to make time for those big, important chats in the morning instead of at night, honouring her circadian rhythm and higher energy levels in the morning.

Worry, anxiety, high adrenaline and cortisol fuel a sense of arousal. The battle for Roz was the see-saw of exhaustion and arousal every day, which created sleep stress and turbulence in her mind. She learned to dampen her sense of arousal and came out the winner.

ACTION: MAKE A REALISTIC DIGITAL CURFEW CHOICE

As always, you have options here. Try five days of having a whole hour pre-bed completely away from all screens. Or start small with an easy win: try a 15-minute screen curfew and see if you want to build up to 30 minutes and then one hour.

If you are really serious about sleep health and well-being, another simple step is to charge your smartphone and let it have a sleepover in a room other than your bedroom. Just as we change our clothes or derobe when we get ready for bed, why don't we do the same with our screen habits – set them down, take them off?

By doing this you widen the pathway towards greater sleep quality and give yourself more opportunity for restful sleep – every night. In turn, having this protective time helps build your social connections away from screens.

What comes up for you? Notice if this makes you feel uneasy or if you want to go all-in and see for yourself how huge the sleep health benefit is when you remove the screen habit from your sleep space. Do what you can to move towards reframing the evening time as a lovely shift into recovery.

If you can commit to this every day for the next few weeks, it will become another everyday Sleep Reset habit. If you would like further guidance on how to lock in this new Reset tool, download my 'Ten steps to a digital curfew' PDF from my website: www.mindtonicsleep.com.

THE HIDDEN COST OF SCREENS

Another reason that I protect at least one hour before we head to bed is the other effects of screens. Do you ever find yourself unconsciously holding your breath when you look at your screen, watch TV or mindlessly scroll TikTok? This is because of 'screen apnoea' (similar to the sleep disorder sleep apnoea - see page 222). Research has shown that looking at small screens is directly linked to sleep health as it creates poor posture and coaches in us a shallower mouth breathing pattern that doesn't send relaxation signals to our nervous system.[32]

Chronic daily micro breath-holds can fuel tiny stresses to your mind and body. These unintentional breath-holds can cause the brain to believe it's on stress standby mode all day long.

Check in with yourself, even now, reading this book. Are your shoulders hunched? Now imagine yourself hunched over in bed at night with a bent neck looking at a small screen. Studies have shown that around 80 per cent of us might be holding our breath or breathing shallowly while looking at a screen.[33]

Social media use has also been linked to increased anxiety, depression and stealing sleep opportunities as well as creating sleep disruption through the night with a decrease in sleep quality.[34]

If you have to work late or don't have the luxury of planning your life in a way that optimises sleep, do the following just before bed:

- untense and unclench

- breathe deeply to avoid unconsciously holding your breath while scrolling

- protect your well-being by taking regular eye breaks

- try blue-light-blocking glasses, which have been proven to be really beneficial (see Resources, page 268).[35] We need to be sleep-smart around technology and also protect eye health

The simple fact is that blue light is all around, but it doesn't need to hold you back. If you can incorporate these simple steps into your evening routine, the timing, quality and duration of your sleep will all improve. In one teen study alone, one hour less phone time equated to one-quarter of a sleep cycle extra each night.[36] Across the week and cumulatively each month and season, that is huge!

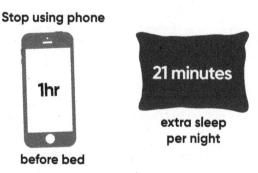

Stop using phone

1hr

before bed

21 minutes

extra sleep per night

While some aspects of this blue-light spectrum have a dark side that is thought to disrupt our performance beyond sleep and impact our mental well-being, it does also have some useful properties, such as being helpful for those suffering from depression.[37] (In clinic, this simply means that we consider the timing and dose of dark and blue light to help reset their sleep.)

Dim the overhead lights

Another simple Sleep Reset step you can take is to try to move away from bright artificial light at night and stay in dim or dark lighting as best and as safely as you can.

The great news is that with a switch to red warm lights at

night, we can enjoy the sense of an evening and social connection without messing up our sleep hormones as red light doesn't disrupt circadian rhythm or melatonin. Candlelight is also amazing at invoking a relaxed, naturally calming mood.

Why don't you also consider the light in your bathroom? Often this is not carefully designed for sleep well-being, yet it is the last room many of us habitually spend time in before bed and is often lit with bright LEDs or a very harsh overhead light.

Could you get a dimmer switch or make some small, subtle changes like choosing to have a shower or clean your teeth at night by candlelight or using a nightlight instead? This easy shift is incredibly effective and works really well to initiate sleep. I have a colour-changing lamp (see Resources, page 269) that I use in my bedroom too. So many of my clients find this one an instant game changer and something they can easily remember that doesn't take much effort.

ACTION: RE-EXAMINE YOUR ROUTINE

This is your opportunity to make some easy changes to your daily routine and existing habits to aid sleep. Given what you have learned about the power of light, consider what changes you could make to your daily routine to help foster better sleep.

- What's my ideal morning routine to ultimately help support my bedtime Sleep Reset?

- How does light help me focus in the day and does it help me sleep better?

- What time could I get up to make the most of the morning light?

- What small change can I make in the morning to harness the health benefits of daylight?

- What change can I easily make at home to ensure a lower light intensity in the evening?

- What is the easiest thing I can do for myself every day, even on challenging days?

- How can I embed some protective time as a new Sleep Reset habit? What would be more useful than slumping in front of the TV or multiple screens?

UNDERSTANDING HOW YOUR SLEEP CHANGES THROUGHOUT THE NIGHT

Sleep is a very active process. Every night, your brain experiences many different stages of sleep, each with a unique sleep ID; each sleep cycle lasts for around 90 minutes and has its own distinctive sleep architecture. The brain waves completely change as we cycle through different depths of sleep and back up to the surface again – a bit like waves across an ocean.[38]

Slow-wave sleep (SWS)

In order to begin the process of sleep, our core body temperature has to dip. After we transition down into sleep, our sleep cycle begins with predominantly slow-wave or deep-wave (non-rapid eye movement, or NREM) sleep.[39]

REM sleep

As the night progresses into the early hours, we go into lighter, more creative REM sleep, which is crucial for emotional well-being. During REM sleep, the sleeping brain wave activity changes and, as our closed eyes move around, we experience lots of dream-processing sleep. This sleep is implicated in longevity, learning and memory consolidation. REM sleep plays a vital role in sorting through our emotions and also enjoys a star turn in our mental health.

A good night's sleep can help your brain press the play, rewind, pause and erase buttons. Researchers believe that, during the slow-wave and deep sleep stages, our brain does some heavy lifting – sorting memories, improving and strengthening them.[40] REM, or the early-hour dream sleep, moves these memories from information to understanding, insight and emotional creativity. This is a time of active recovery for the brain. Masako Tamaki, a researcher at Brown University in Rhode Island, found that neuro-plasticity increases during non-REM sleep and that REM sleep helps protect learning before sleep from being overwritten by sub-sequent information.[41]

THE MYTH OF THE ALL-NIGHTER

We have all been tempted in the past to 'pull an all-nighter' as a big deadline or exam approaches. When I work with schools doing my sleep roadshow, I like to bust the myth that doing so will make you more productive. Quite simply, pulling an all-nighter shuts down your memory 'inbox' and impairs cognition.[42]

Research showed that those who enjoyed a full night of sleep displayed healthy brain patterns related to learning activity. In contrast, those who were sleep-deprived had barely any significant signalling in that region. It was as if the memory and learning files were somehow being missed and any new incoming files were just not able to stick. The brain's brilliant processing system had slowed down and glitched, meaning that any learning was not properly filed or accessible.[43]

As tempting as it is with deadlines approaching, it's good to remember that making time to sleep is always going to help you be more productive.[44]

Discovering the power of your sleep stage cycles

As we've seen, your sleeping brain goes into two distinct states: NREM sleep and REM sleep, and broadly cycles through four sleep stages, ideally in four to five full sleep cycles each night, but every night will be different.

Sleep stages

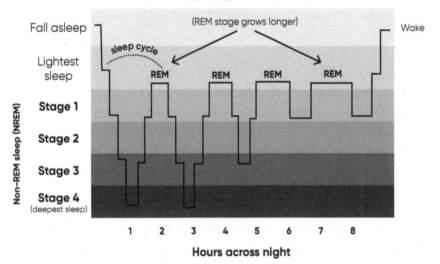

Lightest sleep

We all experience this typical transition from wakefulness – a sensation of sinking down or drifting into sleep that generally only lasts for a few minutes. Key features of this lightest stage of sleep include feeling as if we are neither awake nor asleep and we can respond easily to our environment. In this stage, it's easy to perceive that you are not yet actually asleep. This is because light sleep involves shifts in your consciousness – a wind-down in both body and overall muscle tone and a helpful drop in your core body temperature to help you access your sleep system and start the cycles.

Stage 1: light NREM sleep

This is one of the cool short transition stages before you enter deep sleep. A key feature of this sleep is that the body settles into a state of deep relaxation. There are little bursts of electrical activity in the brain that are important for neuroplasticity and consolidating learning. During this stage, our body continues to wind down, with our heartbeat and breathing slowing down further. We don't tend to experience eye movements in this stage, but may have 'hypnagogic' jerks (sudden, involuntary muscle contractions or twitches). This is a really natural feature and nothing to worry about. Our core body temperature also drops at this stage.

Stages 2–4: SWS, NREM

During these stages, your heart rate and respiration slow dramatically. It is much more difficult be woken up from deep SWS, and your body is fully relaxed with your heartbeat and breathing at their slowest rate. There are no eye movements during this stage and tissue repair and growth and cell regeneration occur, as well as strengthening of our immune system.

These are super-restorative stages of sleep where your brain goes through an active clean-up and renewal – imagine lots of brain rebuilding and DIY. These big SWS processes are naturally timed to happen in the first third of your night.

REM sleep (dream sleep)

Overnight we spend approximately 25 per cent of our total time asleep in REM sleep.[45] Your sleep system takes care of this for you, so you don't have to worry about trying to control it. A key feature of REM sleep is that we are safely 'temporarily paralysed' so that we don't act out our dreams, though lots of eye and eyelid activity still happens.

Many people think that we just have huge chunks of deep sleep and, later on in the night, REM sleep. But actually a little bit of REM occurs in each cycle. This is incredibly reassuring to know when people get stressed over tracking their sleep with wearables and panic that they're not getting the best sleep quality.

MEET THE BLUE SPOT

Did you know that when we go to sleep this super-cool part of the brain - the locus coeruleus, which in Latin means 'blue spot' - slows down and the only time it switches off is during REM sleep periods?

During the day, the blue spot is part of your brain's stress and mobilising response and releases the brain's version of adrenaline – the neurotransmitter noradrenaline (aka norepinephrine). Only in REM sleep does this stay helpfully silent, helping us to refresh and emotionally regulate.

Each of these cycles of sleep is precious even if, at the moment, you only seem to be getting a few cycles at best, or if you are waking up in the middle of the night.

ALL SLEEP COUNTS, NO MATTER WHAT THE NIGHT MAY BRING.

Your inner thermostat

Not many people realise that core body temperature also follows its own circadian rhythm, meaning that it rises and falls across the day and night. This is hugely important for good sleep well-being.

At night, your brain acts as an inner thermostat and your core body temperature needs to drop between 1 and 3°C for your body to go into a sleeping state. Our sleep is particularly sensitive to ambient temperature in our bedroom, so if our temperature rises by more than 3°C, we are more likely to wake up. Every morning, before you wake, the CAR effect (see page 70) works in harmony with this inner thermostat to raise your temperature, bringing you out of sleep. In a nutshell, your body temperature needs to dip as you go off to sleep each night and warm up as you wake up in the morning.

ACTION: PRACTISE CURIOSITY

- Ask yourself how this science-based understanding of the different stages of sleep sits with you.

- Is this a helpful way you can learn to influence everyday well-being? How and why?

- What values does sleep align with for you?

- Think about what you can tweak: what sparked an easy win for you? Your answer will be a helpful jumping-off point to uncover more about your sleep health.

THE THREE MAIN PHASES OF YOUR DAY

Morning: this is the beginning of the cycle. The body decreases the release of melatonin and increases the secretion of cortisol to help you rise up into the morning. At this phase, blood pressure also rises sharply, preparing the body to start the day and propel you into action and the task modes of being awake and alert. That regular wake-up time will help you set your sleep well-being in motion and help you sleep better tonight in terms of both quality and duration.

Midday: the mind and body have the best coordination and cardiovascular activity at this time, which can also contribute to greater muscle strength and faster reaction times. This is a great time to move, seek your exercise or engage in important cognitive tasks. This is followed by a natural recovery period - the post-lunch afternoon dip, your inbuilt nudge to take a rest/ recover.

9-11pm: this is often the very end of the wake cycle and natural alertness, leading down into sleep system transition. Melatonin production increases in response to the onset of darkness, signalling the body to prepare us for sleep. We can very often sense a final energy flush - a nudge of wakefulness - within one to two hours of bedtime. This is naturally inbuilt. I like to see this as a nudge for good sleep well-being and human connection, not energy for scrolling or engaging with more blue-light technology.

SOCIAL JET LAG

Are you familiar with 'social jet lag'? This weekly habit may be sneakily challenging your sleep health. Social jet lag occurs when we go to bed later and wake up later at the weekend than on weekdays and can really impact our mood and well-being.

Super-late nights and chaotic sleep patterns stress your sleep and body clocks internally, just like plane travel across time zones. The Monday 'lag' is very often a result of confusing your body clock over the weekend. Lots of research points to social jet lag being associated with worse mood and greater levels of sleepiness and fatigue.[46] Back in 2006 researchers who coined the term even went as far as to say, 'Social jet lag promotes practically everything that's bad in our bodies.'[47]

Like travel jet lag, social jet lag is a consequence of two competing time zone rhythms inside our brain and body, even if we haven't actually travelled anywhere. It is estimated that two-thirds of us experience at least one hour of social jet lag a week, and a third experience two hours or more – the equivalent to flying from London to the Med and back each week.[48]

Almost all the hormones in our body are on some sort of circadian rhythm and when we shift our sleep and wake-up times, the entire system won't work as efficiently as it could. Choosing a consistent wake-up time can be a powerful way to shift your sleep health.

Choose a consistent wake-up time

This next potent Sleep Reset cue seems so simple, but very often at the beginning of resetting our sleep or trying to solve insomnia it can feel like one of the most challenging.

Getting up at a regular time is so important for sleep well-being. Initially, this is even more helpful than a strict bedtime. Try as best you can to stick within one hour of this for the next two to five weeks. You will be amazed at how quickly your sleep quality improves and you feel refreshed.

For me, this now looks like a habitual wake-up time of 6am, which suits most days and allows me to have some me-time before my teens wake up at the weekend.

What could your average wake-up time be? Choose a time you can commit to and very quickly your inbuilt sleep system will work behind the scenes to get you to wake up and help you feel alert, especially if you also get a healthy dose of morning light.

'But I'll miss my snoozing!' I hear you cry. This small, powerful step is very often met with resistance or a litany of excuses: 'I can't because ...', 'I feel too tired', 'I can't imagine doing that because I am not a morning person'. What is the first excuse that comes to YOUR mind?

By overcoming the obstacles in your mind and choosing to adopt this for now (maybe not forever) you can work with your inner sleep tech in the fastest way possible, giving it the biological cues it needs to synch wake and sleep cycles for you. This week's 'Deep Sleep Ease' audio tool (page 95) helps coach your unconscious habits and make this easy to do.

In a nutshell, the timing of morning light in harmony with the biological 'shower' of cortisol and adrenaline is easily the most important cue for sleep health and well-being, followed by prioritising a regular wake-up time.

UNDERSTANDING YOUR CHRONOTYPE

Your chronotype refers to your individual preferences when it comes to waking and sleeping, including the time of day you are most alert and at your personal best – the pattern of your instinctive sleep-wake cycle. We all have a genetic component to our individual chronotypes,[49] but whether we consider ourselves a morning (lark) type, an evening (owl) type or a neutral type can also depend on the following factors:

- our biological sex and chronotype

- our current age and the life stages of puberty, pregnancy, midlife, perimenopause, menopause and older age, all of which can nudge our chronotype around

- our exposure to environmental light

- our work patterns

- our sleep behaviours

It's really easy to work out your natural sleep preference (your personal chronotype). In clinic, I use a simple quiz based on the Morningness-Eveningness Questionnaire. This is a set of questions that ask you to note the time when you have your best energy, your mealtime preferences, what time you like to do some work and exercise, and what time you would go to bed and wake if you were to sleep over the course of a week without setting an alarm. You can ask yourself similar questions to identify what time of day you are at your personal best. (If you want to take the chronotype quiz, please go to my website: www.mindtonicsleep.com.) In reality, most people are already aware of whether they are a 'morning person', a 'night owl' or not bothered either way without answering these questions.

Identifying your chronotype can help you stay as best you can in a rhythm with your sleep health. I help people advocate in workplace settings to, where possible, match their working hours or deep concentration work hours with their best energy. It's so beneficial if you can work with your natural energy and not fuel fatigue. And remember, regardless of chronotype, we all experience that mid-afternoon dip in energy based on our inner sleep systems. Your chronotype can become a helpful clue as to when to do your best work, when to schedule rest and when to use your sleep tools as appropriate for you.

Whatever your chronotype, becoming more aware of the benefits of natural light mornings, brightly lit workspace days and dimmer, darker evenings will greatly influence your sleep health.

ALWAYS TRY TO WORK WITH RATHER THAN AGAINST YOUR NATURAL BODY CLOCK. DOING THIS CAN HELP YOU STAY IN BALANCE.

Learning about the importance of light was pivotal in helping my client Suki overcome a six-month episode of chronic insomnia. Suki had experienced fragile sleep for most of her life. Staying asleep was a challenge and, when I met her, she was desperate to find a solution that didn't involve more expensive gimmicks and pills. Having white-knuckled it through insomnia by intermittently taking sleeping tablets, she no longer wanted to rely on medication and craved some semblance of sleep balance.

Suki had no idea about the influence of light on sleep and, within two weeks of getting out into early-morning light, she shifted from three hours to five or six hours of sleep a night, which gave her the energy and focus to embark on her goal of engaging in a daily mind–body strength-training habit. Suki also specifically chose a consistent wake-up time of 6am across seven days to coach her body clock into a new pattern.

Welcome to a new world of choices and habits you can more easily make now that you know the science behind sleep and have a better understanding of the day and night cycle and how to work with, not against, it. That's the exciting part of this story – most of us have control over when we open our curtains in the morning and put down our phones and turn off the lights at night, so you can embark on supporting sleep health right now.

In Week 3, you will discover how nutrition can benefit your sleep health.

WEEK 2 SLEEP RESET TOOLKIT

Last week we built your new sleep mindset and paved the way for sleep success with the foundation tools for your new approach to sleep, priming a healthy self-awareness and practical action approach. We didn't rush into changing too much or using fast fixes; instead we built a sleep-kind, feel-good way of thinking.

This week, you can choose to harness brilliant circadian science with a new layer of easy, realistic, short sleep-priming tools that work from morning to night. If you can, stay with the tools from Week 1, layering this week's practices on top.

YOUR WEEK 2 TOOLKIT RECOVERY MENU

1. Your Mindset Tool: Calm Cave Focus (5-minute guided audio download)

2. Your Breathing Tool: Your Big Five Energy (5-minute guided audio download)

3. Your Sleep Hypnosis: Deep Sleep Ease (7-minute guided audio download)

Quick cheat sheet

Before we get started with this week's tools, let's make sure you're priming your inner sleep tech and doing the basics really well:

The power of sleep timing

Anchor in your sleep health from morning to night-time:

- AM: choose the most realistic consistent wake-up time that you can stick to for at least five mornings of the week (ideally seven as we're teaching your circadian clocks to synch up).

- PM: choose your best bedtime – a time that gifts you the best opportunity for adequate, good sleep.
- Pause this habit: don't press the snooze button for the next seven days.

The power of light and dark
- Seek morning light upon waking: really harness the power of light across that first phase of your day.
- Screen-protect your sleep: blue light at night is generally a big challenge for your inner sleep tech. Start with 15 minutes away from screens and blue light before bed and build up to a protective hour to make sleep quality gains.
- Try the new sleep health habit of a weekend morning visualisation instead of hitting the snooze button. This will help you avoid social jet lag and steer you away from the autopilot weekday habit of doomscrolling.

By making sure you have the Sleep Reset circadian principles covered, you can layer up your Sleep Reset with this week's audio tools, which will give you practical tweaks to help supercharge your sleep recovery day and night so you can:

- enhance your morning to boost sleep quality tonight
- have extra support when unwinding before bed
- leave behind the battle with your snooze button
- choose to become more of a morning person and get the most out of your day
- leave behind tiredness
- . . . or just simply choose to look after your sleep in the most realistic way you can

For over a decade I've been sharing that sleep starts the moment you wake up – and this week you get to experience what this feels like in your life. You can better connect to your inner sleep technology in a realistic way. The audio tools this week will help you turn the tide and get back in circadian harmony.

Your Mindset Tool: Calm Cave Focus

This quick tool is for every one of us who naturally experiences momentarily waking up too early or in the middle of the night. This is a brilliant in-the-moment tool that, when practised regularly, offers you a restful choice if you don't want to keep getting out of bed and waking others, if it's too chilly or if you would like to practise enjoying an opportunity to rest as best you can even when your sleep is on pause.

This tool will help you calm down your racing mind and shift into rest mode. It will show you how to switch from awake to active rest in the middle of the night or in the early hours.

With this exercise you flex your sensory muscles away from the planning or worry modes that are so prevalent at night and choose bed rest over bed stress.

Your Breathing Tool: Your Big Five Energy

This is an energising wake-up tool that allows you to power up your day in the right way (and is a simple alternative to hitting the snooze button!).

In this breathing exercise, you practise ways to stay away from runaway cortisol and it helps create a helpful space for you to choose your daytime habits with more intention and care.

Practising this as a daytime approach helps create harmony later on for your sleep health. This daytime habit will also become your ally any time you wake up too early or want to connect with better energy quickly.

Your Sleep Hypnosis: Deep Sleep Ease

This week we're going to deepen your sleep with another themed audio download that will help you build that easier sleep connection.

This week's hypnosis has a really nice twist, starting with a deep sleep body scan and moving into a hypnosis visualisation that makes your sleep time a whole lot easier.

The skill you build on here is designed to help you instil a consistent way to begin resting your body on command – an essential building block for your Sleep Reset.

MAKING BIG DEEP SLEEP GAINS

I love sharing a study by Maren J. Cordi and her colleagues that demonstrates just how highly effective hypnosis is at increasing deep or slow wave sleep (SWS).[50] After participants listened to the hypnotic suggestion to 'sleep deeper', subsequent SWS increased by 81 per cent and time spent awake was reduced by 67 per cent.

Listening to this unique guided audio allows you to embed the insights you've learned in this chapter and to imagine more easily responding to the seasons and taking those steps to protect yourself from any blue light or other evening habits that may be holding you back.

The transcript is hosted on www.mindtonicsleep.com.

YOUR WEEK 2 BONUS TOOLS

Think in ink

For me, this practical tool is a neat way to shift my focus and dial down my day in a calmer way. It's an easy habit that helps focus on evening recovery rather than continuous planning.

In the early evening, create a moment to get what's in your head down onto the page. Take a notepad and split the page into three:

- PLACE IT: on the left-hand side, place big troubles and tiny troubles. Try to keep your mind focused on the day that has just passed and the next day only.
- PLAN IT: on the right-hand side, match each point you've just written with what you can change and influence, what you can accept and what you will address this week. Embrace self-kindness when doing this.
- PARK IT: put it all away with a simple 'That's enough for now' sidenote to yourself.

Top tip: keep the notepad away from your bedside table. Get into a new habit (just like with your phone – see page 78) of placing it out of arm's reach so you can truly disconnect from what is on your list. But, of course, the choice is yours.

Timing is everything here. Ideally across the weeks you can slide this worry-time habit further away from sleep time and make it count. There is a big difference between healthy planning and unhealthy worries. When you understand that, it's game-changing and can be really helpful when it comes to looking after your sleep health.

You can download a 'Place it, plan it, park it' sheet from www. mindtonicsleep.com.

Make a self-celebration note

You've now got two weeks of practising a new sleep-kind mindset under your belt! How could you best acknowledge your success? Aside from a mental note, think about the way you want to track your progress. You can scribble in the back of this book or deep-dive into personal journalling. There's also a Sleep Success Tracker on my website that provides some useful tried-and-tested prompts and is a lovely way of documenting your personal Sleep Reset (see www.mindtonicsleep.com).

YOUR REALISTIC SLEEP RESET 'PRESCRIPTION'

This week, I want you to build your own Sleep Reset prescription. Think about your favourite tool from last week. What really resonated with you? Begin the week by layering in your favourite tool and then, each day, add in the mindset, breathing or sleep hypnosis tools from this week. Get super creative, slot them in your diary and give yourself some easy reminders. Starting in the early working week is a realistic way to give your sleep health that VIP care it needs. What could this look like for you?

Tool	Monday	Tuesday	Wednesday	Thursday	Friday	Saturday (optional)	Sunday
Mindset							
Breathing							
Sleep Hypnosis							

If this self-directed planning feels a little too much, you can download a prescription for each week from my website: www.mindtonicsleep.com.

WEEK 3: FUELLING YOUR SLEEP WELL-BEING

Welcome to the midway point of the Sleep Reset! By now, you will hopefully be noticing real, beneficial change in your relationship to your sleep. You've done a lot of hard work in the previous two weeks. This week we'll discover the impact of nutrition on your sleep health before we deep dive into combating sleep stress in Week 4.

In my experience, once people have got on board with their mindset, updated their sleep story (see page 40) and explored circadian science, it can feel energising and they get a thirst for how else they can help themselves. One of the most frequent questions I am asked is what the impact of food and nutrition is on sleep. As we all know, nutrition is really complex and individualised, but this week I seek to share some of the lesser-known and exciting discoveries in the world of sleep health and offer you some evidence-based ways to fuel and protect your long-term sleep health.

This week will help you understand how the architecture of your sleep is subtly but powerfully supported and influenced by what you consume during the day, inspiring you to make your own choices. This is what I call a 360-degree approach to your Sleep Reset.

EVERY DAY YOU FUEL YOUR BRAIN AND SLEEP HEALTH BY WHAT YOU CHOOSE TO EAT AND THE TIMING OF YOUR MEALS.

HOW SLEEP AFFECTS OUR APPETITE

In the past decade, we have learned an enormous amount about the relationship between lack of sleep and its effects on appetite, obesity and weight gain, as well as its impact on insulin resistance and glucose regulation. There is substantial research to prove that short or disturbed sleep increases our appetite for high-calorie foods.[1]

Missed sleep certainly skews our cravings for ultra-processed foods (UPFs). As sleep also controls glucose production, short or missed sleep initiates an unhelpful blood sugar rollercoaster in our body, sending our hormone balance haywire and massively altering our appetite.

Why does blood sugar control matter?

Good blood sugar control is important for your health and your sleep well-being. Did you know that blood sugar stability is related to everything from influencing our hormones and whether we feel energised or fatigued all the way through to how well we can fall asleep and stay asleep?

Your sleep at night is really sensitive to blood sugar disruptions. Recent studies show that 80 per cent of people who don't have diabetes still experience glucose spikes every day.[2]

Glucose spikes can affect your focus and health behaviours, and fuel the cortisol arc that is so unhelpful to sleep. Glucose spikes also have a direct impact on our hunger hormone levels. The more spikes we experience, the more swings in hunger we get – we go from eating a meal to being extremely hungry again in an hour or two, instead of being full for hours.

There are two hormones responsible for controlling hunger, appetite and satiety:

- Ghrelin stimulates appetite, making you hungry and crave food, which is why it's known as the hunger hormone.

- Leptin is its opposite number – the hormone that makes you feel full and sated.

In those with healthy overnight sleep, these two hormones are best buddies and work in perfect harmony to regulate normal feelings of hunger and appetite. However, leptin seemingly falls off the map when we are sleep-deprived.

The stress of missed sleep or fewer than four hours a night creates a 'hangry' panic mode of calorie-laden sugar cravings. Why? You've guessed it – ghrelin levels go up and leptin levels go down, leading to increased appetite and food intake and less satisfaction with the food already consumed.

An interesting study at Stanford University discovered that just one night of sleep deprivation and poor sleep can lead to a severe suppression of leptin levels.[3] Another US study by sleep researchers showed that one night of poor-quality sleep can lead to a 20 per cent increase in ghrelin levels.[4]

Indeed, research has shown that sleep-deprived adults tend to have higher ghrelin levels, more hunger and experience fewer feelings of fullness compared to adults who get seven to nine hours of sleep a night.[5] This perfect storm of increased waking hours, frustration and tiredness creates an opportunity to overestimate your nutrition needs, fuelling a tendency to overeat. In simple terms, this means we carry on consuming surplus calories with a tendency towards starchy, salty, crunchy, sugary snacks.[6]

In one study, more than 4,000 people reported the amount of sleep they got each night.[7] Those who got fewer than six hours were twice as likely to have cells that were less sensitive to insulin or to have full-blown diabetes. This was true even after the researchers took other lifestyle habits into account.

If you have blood sugar levels that are either too high or too low overnight, you may find yourself tired through the next day. Lethargy and insomnia can both have their roots in blood sugar control, which can be the key to re-establishing a healthy sleep pattern.

High blood sugar levels can impact your sleep – the more sugar you eat during the day, the more likely it is you'll wake up during the night (we see the same impact with sugary alcohol). It could be that the high sugar levels make it less comfortable for you to sleep – it may make you feel too warm, or irritable and unsettled. Low blood glucose levels (hypoglycaemia) can also have a negative impact on your sleep. If you are taking insulin or other blood sugar medication, you may be at risk of low blood sugar levels during the night, which can disrupt your sleep pattern and lead to difficulty waking in the morning and tiredness through the day.

Another factor is the need to go to the toilet excessively during the night, which can be a symptom of high blood sugar. This can have a pronounced impact on the ability to get a good night's sleep.

If you have diabetes, too little sleep negatively affects every area of your management, including how much you eat, what you choose to eat, how you respond to insulin and your mental health. If you get fewer than six hours of sleep per night regularly, your diabetes will be harder to manage.

Proper sleep well-being and daytime rest isn't just important for your diabetes management – it may also put you in a better mood and give you more energy to engage with your life.

Of course, it goes without saying that UPFs and high-sugar foods really do have a big impact on our sleep well-being close to bedtime, so the more you can cut down on these, the better.

REGULAR GREAT SLEEP LEADS TO BETTER BLOOD SUGAR CONTROL THE NEXT DAY, WHEREAS POOR SLEEP LEADS TO LARGER SPIKES IN BLOOD SUGAR.

I am not here to prescribe your food or nutrition choices, but I am here to share the sleep-related research that may inform your personal sleep well-being. I feel it's a more refreshing approach to look at what you can add in rather than give you a list of what you shouldn't do.

ACTION: WHY NOT TRY A POST-DINNER STROLL?

After-supper strolls boost heart health, as any movement does, but they also reduce the blood sugar spikes that accompany large meals. Several studies have found that a short walk after eating helps regulate blood glucose levels, making it particularly effective for anyone with diabetes, irritable bowel syndrome (IBS) or inflammatory bowel disease (IBD) as it also creates a break from mindless evening snacking.[8]

Try to move your muscles for ten minutes after lunch and dinner – walk around the block, go up and down the stairs a few times or do some energetic housework. Move within 90 minutes of the end of your meal to see an effect on your glucose levels. This is particularly powerful in helping with the post-meal glucose crash that causes lethargy.

Other positive side effects of a post-meal evening walk include the release of serotonin, part of our sleep-promoting story, as well as lower stress and better digestion. Just as early-morning light boosts your sleep, so does an evening stroll, particularly at sunset, as this later light sends an optimal sleep cue to the sleep sensors (the neurons at the back of our eyes that stabilise our body clocks).[9]

Looking at the evening sky or watching the sunset actually reduces and mitigates some of the unhelpful effects of blue light at night. As Dr Andrew Huberman has put it: 'Viewing light circa sunset adjusts the sensitivity of the cells in the eye such that it buffers you against some of the negative effects of light late at night. So, I call it sort of my Netflix vaccination.'[10]

My clients also like the fact that an evening stroll helps them offset some of the blue light of their working day, as it has a protective effect. I find this a particularly popular Sleep Reset habit that people can easily do.

THE LINK BETWEEN SLEEP AND WEIGHT

There is no escaping the fact that getting little sleep makes it much more challenging to stay within a healthy body weight range and if, like me, you have polycystic ovary syndrome (PCOS), then sleep is extremely important for balancing hormones and maintaining a healthy body composition.[11] Chronic insomnia is also associated with potential fluctuations that drive weight gain.

Lack of sleep affects the parts of our brain responsible for impulse control, potentially leaving us with a reduced desire to eat a balanced diet, further impacting sleep. The great news is that healthy sleep patterns can help promote healthy body composition. Overnight sleep processes play an important role in tissue regeneration and a healthy body composition of bones, fat and muscles.

SLEEP-FRIENDLY NUTRITION

'SIMPLE AND SMALL CHANGES TO IMPROVING YOUR SLEEP CAN HAVE MAJOR IMPACTS ON THE WAY YOUR BODY RESPONDS TO FOOD AND THEREFORE YOUR HEALTH.'

TIM SPECTOR, PROFESSOR OF GENETIC EPIDEMIOLOGY AT KING'S COLLEGE LONDON[12]

Our diet has huge consequences for how well we sleep. Sleep-friendly food is also brain- and gut-friendly food, and a deeper understanding of the ways you can boost your gut health has helped many people to sleep better (more on this on page 113). While nutrition doesn't create sleep, it certainly supports and influences it.

I have many brilliant colleagues in high-performance sports nutrition and one I regularly collaborate with is Kate Shilland, a top nutritionist working with elite athletes and Premier League clubs. Kate has taught me so much and we agree that a nutrition-friendly mindset, which takes a health-kind, unrestrictive and consistent approach to eating, is the first step towards building confidence and good eating habits.

Having a nutrition-friendly mindset means:

- trusting that you can improve your sleep health and performance through the daily food choices you make
- being open to new choices and variety, and being curious to learn what personally works for you
- being honest and kind with yourself about your obstacles and habits and being open to helpful change
- less restriction and shame-related 'bad'/banned food behaviours

Whenever we are making sleep health-related changes, it's always useful to think about healthy whole foods and plants that we can add in, rather than simply focusing on what we want to cut out. This is a far more sustainable approach that excites your motivation and infuses your choices with meaning rather than thinking, *Ugh, I can't have that* or shaming any one food group.

A nutrition-friendly mindset is an approach to eating that focuses on getting the 'good' stuff into our bodies for wider health rather than worrying too much about excluding or cutting out food groups. It is a shift in thinking from deprivation to abundance that can be incredibly liberating, particularly if we have been caught up in a cycle of on-off dieting culture for a long time. Having a focus on a diet mindset often leads to feelings of restriction, guilt, self-loathing and even anxiety. The opposite of this is a self-compassionate Sleep Reset approach.

Thinking in this nutrition-friendly way goes a long way to

improving your sleep quality and, during the daytime, helps you with blood sugar regulation and focus.

A large body of literature supports the hypothesis that there is a beneficial link between what we eat and our sleep well-being.[13] Specifically, we are beginning to uncover a strong association between sleep and diet quality, possibly via changes in neuro-inflammation and neurogenesis (our brain's plasticity).

Eating plant-based foods, including vegetables, grains, nuts, seeds, legumes and fruits, influences our sleep quality and supports our mental health.

Studies show that the nutritional quality of your food through-out the day makes a difference at night.[14] The more calories you get from UPFs high in sugar and saturated fat, the more likely you are to experience sleep disturbances. On the other hand, diets high in fibre, nutrient-dense plants and lean protein seem to help you fall asleep and stay asleep throughout the night.

My intention is to never tell you exactly how and what to eat – my five-week sleep method is all about creating sleep health that is unique to you, and this also links to diet. However, I would like to share with you some foods that have been shown to be help-ful in promoting better sleep:

The superstar foods for better sleep

It's always beneficial to include as many whole foods and plant-based nutrients (fruit, vegetables, nuts, seeds, whole grains and legumes) as possible in your diet to support your sleep well-being. By all means start small and aim for five a day before challenging yourself to add one extra each day for seven days.

Over and over, studies show that a higher dietary intake of plants and whole foods and certain polyphenols may be potentially associated with better sleep quality.[15] Polyphenols are a type of antioxidant found in certain foods and beverages, including black tea.

THE POWER OF WHOLEGRAINS

Wholegrains such as oats, brown rice and wholewheat bread are better for your sleep compared to their white counterparts because these wholegrain foods undergo less processing, and so they retain more health benefits.

Essential nutrients for sleep contained in wholegrains such as potassium, magnesium and calcium are stripped from the grains when they are processed from brown rice to white rice, wholewheat to white flour, and so on.

Tryptophan-rich foods

Tryptophan is an amino acid that increases the production of sleep-promoting neurotransmitters. Choose to add tryptophan-rich foods to your diet to help promote sleep. The best sources are turkey, eggs, dairy, tofu and nuts and seeds (see pages 114–115) Cashews, almonds and pistachios contain tryptophan as well as being rich in calcium and magnesium (you'll hear more about magnesium on page 117).

Calcium- and protein-rich foods support the conversion of tryptophan into sleep-triggering melatonin, while magnesium calms the body and relaxes muscles. My favourite mid-evening snack is honey on sourdough toast because carbohydrate-containing foods help the tryptophan-rich ingredients get absorbed by the brain.[16]

Omega-3s

Omega-3 fats are a group of fats we need to stay healthy, and they are especially good for sleep, brain and heart health. Recent research shows that low levels of omega-3 are linked to lower levels of melatonin and poorer sleep duration, and studies in both children and adults reveal that supplementing your diet with omega-3 actually increases sleep duration and sleep quality.[17]

New research suggests that omega-3 fatty acid levels are associated with healthy sleep duration. In one study, people who regularly underslept (five hours habitually) had lower levels of omega-3 than those who regularly got adequate sleep (seven hours habitually).[18]

A 2014 study showed that eating oily fish seems to have a positive impact on sleep efficiency and daily function after sleep.[19] Another study suggests that vitamin D and omega-3 fatty acids can also increase the feel-good hormone serotonin.[20] Higher levels of omega-3 in our diet are certainly associated with better sleep.[21]

The three main omega-3 fatty acids are:

- eicosapentaenoic acid (EPA)
- docosahexaenoic acid (DHA)
- alpha-linolenic acid (ALA)

EPA and DHA mainly come from animal foods, predominantly oily fish, whereas ALA is mostly found in plant oils and natural seeds.

Oily fish is the best source of omega-3 fats, though it is also found in:

- some oils including flax (also known as flaxseed oil and linseed oil), walnut, soya, pumpkin and algae
- green leafy vegetables, such as spinach and broccoli
- nuts, especially walnuts
- seeds, especially flax (linseed), pumpkin, chia and hemp
- wild rice
- seaweed and algae
- edamame beans
- spirulina

To get more of these into your diet, try sprinkling flaxseed over your porridge and cereals, or nuts and seeds over your salads.

ACTION: UP YOUR OMEGA-3 INTAKE

Aim to eat two portions of fish per week, at least one of which should be oily. A portion is 140g, but you could have two or three smaller portions throughout the week. All oily fish contains omega-3 fats. You can choose from fresh, tinned or frozen fish. Sardines are a brilliant low-cost and tinned option - these small oily fish pack a real flavour punch, with just one tin providing around 2.7g of omega-3.

Some foods - such as eggs or even some frozen fish - have omega-3 fats added to them.

If your family, like mine, are not so keen on oily fish, ensure you take a high-quality omega-3 supplement to add in some extra support as it's so important for brain, gut and especially women's sleep health (see Resources, page 265). If you are vegan or vegetarian, you can take marine oils made from algae.

Protein

Daily dietary protein plays an important role in recovery and growth, but is also now in the sleep well-being spotlight. We already know that, in general, diets rich in fibre, fruits, vegetables and anti-inflammatory nutrients and lower in saturated fat (for example, the Mediterranean diet) are associated with better sleep quality. But there is now a proven link between diets higher in protein and better sleep quality.[22]

Looking at the sleep literature, there is no doubt that making sure you have daily protein is amazing for many things, especially brain and sleep health. Protein seems to help you fall asleep faster and plays a role in promoting good sleep health. Studies have shown that dietary protein intake was associated with sleep duration, quality and patterns – dietary protein does indeed help build healthy sleep.[23] A study of over 4,500 non-shift workers found that a low daily percentage of protein (less than 16 per cent) was associated with insomnia and poor-quality sleep, whereas having more than 19 per cent daily protein was linked to maintaining good sleep. A general guide I share with my clients – and something that I aim for in midlife – is to think about having 20 per cent protein daily for better sleep health. Do research the Reference Nutrient Intake for your own body composition.

Pro- and prebiotics

Looking after your complete gut health by including probiotics and prebiotics in your diet is beneficial for brain function and over-all health. While it's easy to get confused between probiotics and prebiotics, the main takeaway here is to think about fuelling your gut microbiome with a variety of choices that suit how you eat. For me, I always start my day with goat's milk kefir, but I also like to add in a variety of both pro- and prebiotics where I can across my week.

Emerging research really zooms in on the direct impact of prebiotics on our sleep quality. This is beautifully highlighted in a University of Colorado study that revealed that prebiotics could have a significant effect on the quality of non-REM and REM sleep, with research proving that we can obtain sleep-supporting nutrients from eating two kiwis an hour before bed.[24]

You'll find probiotics in yoghurt and sauerkraut, while prebi-otics are found in whole grains, walnuts, almonds, bananas, greens, onions, garlic, leeks, soybeans and artichokes. Both probiotics and prebiotics are added to some foods and are also available as dietary supplements.

In the field of nutrition we're beginning to realise what's beneficial for building a healthy brain and therefore healthy sleep health: it comes down to more plants, a diverse wholefood diet and a good proportion of protein.

WHY CHERRIES ARE THE SMART CHOICE

Cherries are one of the few foods that contain a natural source of melatonin, which is key for managing our sleep-wake cycle. One study found that tart cherry juice concentrate was beneficial in managing disturbed sleep, while another, published in the *European Journal of Nutrition*, revealed that drinking tart cherry juice before bed provided small improvements in the duration and quality of sleep in chronic insomnia sufferers.[25]

In a 2018 study, adults who drank tart cherry juice twice a day for seven days slept longer and reported better sleep quality than those who didn't drink the juice, so it could be worth trying if you're looking for ways to ramp up your sleep quality.[26] This study also showed that participants benefited from an extra 84 minutes of sleep time - almost a whole sleep cycle.

Supplements containing cherry juice extract and the amino acid L-theanine also yield good results, with research showing that 200ml of L-theanine can support good sleep while also helping to lower blood pressure.[27] L-theanine (first discovered in green tea - see page 129) has relaxing effects on brain activity during sleep. Multiple studies have found that it seems to produce a calming effect that reduces the time it takes to fall asleep as well as improving sleep quality.[28]

Sleep-friendly foods to consider trying

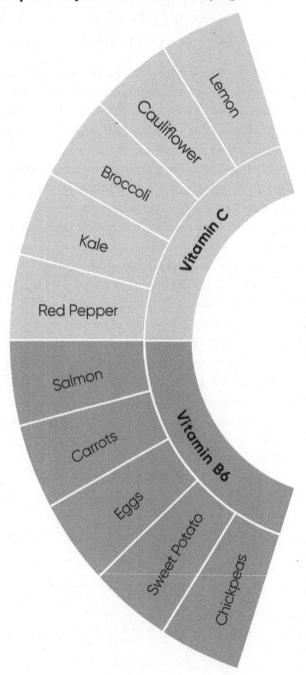

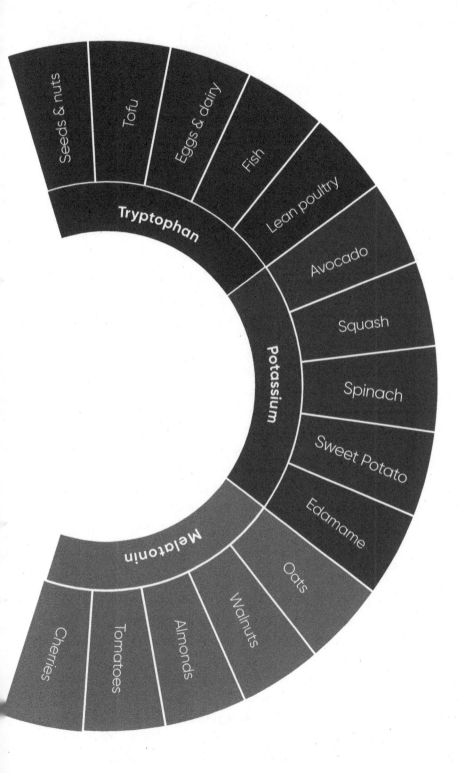

REDISCOVERING MOTHER NATURE'S SLEEP SUPPORTS

You may have come across the well-being pioneer, world-famous naturopath and proponent of mushrooms for health, Dr Andrew Weil. But did you know that mushrooms help sleep health in powerful ways?

Over the last 20 years, science has been waking up to the well-being benefits of mushrooms for brain health and sleep.[29] This is an incredibly exciting new area, and the reishi mushroom in particular has been used for over 4,000 years in Asian medicine as an insomnia sleep aid solution (see Resources, page 270).

Stunning research in 2021 shone a light on how the reishi mushroom exerts an anti-insomnia effect, day and night.[30] The adaptogenic qualities of reishi mushrooms also help to balance levels of stress hormones such as cortisol and adrenaline.

Known in research studies by its full name, *Ganoderma lucidum*, reishi could be a good plant-based natural sleep health aid for your Sleep Reset.

Research shows that, with regular use, consumption of reishi mushrooms can help support quality sleep and deeper sleep.[31] A study published in the *Journal of Ethnopharmacology* found that three days of reishi mushroom use 'significantly increased total sleep time and non-rapid eye movement sleep' (deep sleep).[32]

Over the last few years, it's been easier to source good-quality reishi from trusted sources. If you're curious, like me, and want to see if reishi can be beneficial for your sleep, there are some easy drink blends on the market now. In fact, I've swapped my evening warm drink to a cup of reishi mushroom powder added to a milky tea or plant-based protein smoothie (see Resources, page 270).

There are two other sleep quality superstars on the block: Lactium® and lactoferrin. You can think of these milk proteins as Mother Nature's own potent sleep remedy. Lactium® acts effectively and naturally on the central nervous system, providing a stress reduction effect and helping us transition down into sleep with greater ease. Lactoferrin is an anti-inflammatory protein abundant in human tears, saliva and breast milk. It also plays a starring role in managing stress and supporting sleep health, and research shows that it has a beneficial effect on sleep quality.[33] What I love about the discovery of Lactium® and lactoferrin is that they both provide a holistic sleep aid away from the 'dark' side of sleeping pills and they are natural and safe to use every day to protect our overall sleep health.

Depending on your own medical and health history, are these new discoveries something you can research this week and see if they are right for you?

Supplements for better sleep

Magnesium

Many of my clients aren't aware of the magic of magnesium – it is so much more than just something to add to your bath to repair and relax muscles.

Magnesium is pretty special stuff and is involved in over 600 enzymatic reactions in your body. It affects everything from energy levels to brain function and also serves as a powerful sleep supplement, promoting muscle relaxation, calm and more restorative sleep. Magnesium helps to calm down your thinking by regulating the neurotransmitter known as GABA (an important amino acid that plays a part in your sleep well-being). Deficiencies in GABA are often associated with insomnia and sleep disturbances.

There's no end to magnesium's special powers – it even protects against depression and migraines, and manages the symptoms of anxiety while helping to sensitise cells to the effects of insulin, cutting down on sugar in the blood and reducing stress and inflammation.[34] As we've seen, blood sugar regulation hugely supports sleep health. Late nights and less sleep disrupt our blood sugar the next day so magnesium has a rolling protective effect in many ways.

Essential to your diet, it's the second most common electrolyte in the human body and, in short, it's one of those minerals that pretty much everyone in this high-stress society could benefit from consuming more of.

High-magnesium foods include dark leafy greens, seeds, beans, fish, wholegrains, nuts, dark chocolate, yoghurt, avocados and bananas, but despite being present in many foods, magnesium deficiencies are common. This is largely due to our high-grain diets, which are poor sources of this valuable mineral, and taking a supplement is the most obvious way to maintain good levels.

Low magnesium is often found in people with sleep disorders. In fact, for midlife, one study showed that this was as high as 58 per cent.[35] This is yet more proof of how magnesium plays a starring role in your 360-degree approach to sleep health.[36]

Magnesium threonate is considered the most effective type of magnesium to cross the blood–brain barrier, leading to memory consolidation during sleep and enhancing the ability of the mitochondria – our body's powerhouse cells (or internal batteries), which generate energy – to recharge.[37] It also increases neuroplasticity, aka the brain's ability to grow, change and learn.[38]

CBD

One of the fastest-growing, holistic sleep aids is cannabidiol, more commonly known as CBD. Used in abundance in ancient times, particularly throughout the Indian subcontinent and central Asia, it is widely accepted today as an effective pain reliever and to treat conditions including Parkinson's disease, epilepsy and anxiety.[39]

High-quality CBD has definite benefits for your sleep when used alongside the Sleep Reset.[40] Did you know that the hypothalamus – the peanut-sized structure buried deep in the brain – is actually enriched with cannabinoid receptors and plays an integral role in your circadian rhythm?

Understanding the endocannabinoid system is essential to understanding the effect CBD may have on sleep. Your brilliant endocannabinoid system is a complex neurochemical network in your body that regulates a fascinating multitude of systems, but is especially

linked to pain and sleep. CBD is thought to help people with insomnia because it works with the hypothalamus to regulate stress and
support your sleep–wake system to get back into harmony. It is being
explored in an explosion of high-quality studies for sleep and mental
well-being. Interestingly, cannabinoids reduce activity in the
amygdala – the part of the brain that controls panic reactions, fear and
a deep stress response in the body – and a few studies have found that
cannabinoids reduced nightmares and helped with insomnia.[41]

It's thought that CBD can suppress the dysregulated cycle of
stress hormones, which we so often see in insomnia, and could be a
promising sleep apnoea treatment aid.[42]

I used a high-quality CBD balm and tincture to support my
turbulent sleep while awaiting surgery for my cervical neck injury,
as well as during my six-month healing journey (see Resources,
page 270). I was astounded at how beneficial CBD was for managing intense pain on top of my insomnia.

Vitamin D

Simply put, our sleep health needs daily vitamin D because it helps
us produce melatonin and maintain a healthy circadian rhythm (see
page 65), as well as supporting our immunity, bone and muscle
health. Vitamin D helps us convert timely tryptophan into serotonin
for melatonin – all supportive and essential for sleep well-being.

Vitamin D is both a hormone that is synthesised by sunlight
and a nutrient that we need. A seminal study showed that adequate
vitamin D supplementation boosts sleep duration and quality,
especially in those struggling with sleep.[43] Sleep studies show that
if adults and children are low in vitamin D, they are more likely to
have trouble falling asleep, have poor sleep quality and be prone to
frequent night wakings.[44]

Globally, vitamin D insufficiency is really common, and in the
UK it is one of the most common deficiencies (the latest NHS stats
show that as many as one in five are deficient).[45] Many of us are now
living in urban cities at northern latitudes, working indoors and
accessing less natural daylight. In the UK, the NHS recommends

that we should supplement with vitamin D for half the year in the autumn and winter. Even I've been surprised when blood test results have shown that I'm low in vitamin D as I spend a large proportion of my working life outside.

If you want to make a choice to top up, I always recommend doing so with an easily digestible oral spray, even if you take a multivitamin. Vitamin D is a relatively low-cost health supplement that has so many benefits beyond sleep for mind and body health.

THREE EASY WAYS TO BOOST VITAMIN D

1. Spend more time outside in sunlight.

2. Eat foods rich in vitamin D (oily fish, liver, red meat, egg yolks and fortified dairy and plant milks).

3. Potentially use a vitamin D3 daily top-up, especially in the autumn and winter.

Adding these foods and supplements to your diet forms an integral part of your nutritional approach to sleep health. Increasing omega-3s, tryptophan and plant-based foods also helps you look after your brain and your mental well-being.

RESTING YOUR BONES

Bone density research from the Medical College of Wisconsin found that sleep actually helps build up your bones.[46] Sleep well-being especially plays a protective role in female bone health in midlife. In one study, women who self-reported sleeping five hours or fewer per night had significantly lower bone mineral density at four sites – whole body, hip, neck and spine – compared to women who slept seven hours a night.[47] The difference they observed is equivalent to one year of ageing.

The body undergoes an array of healthy processes during sleep, including growth and repair of our bones, during which old tissue is removed and new bone tissue is formed.

So, what can you do to keep your bones healthy?

- Sleep well regularly for around five sleep cycles per night (see page 87).

- Include plenty of calcium in your diet. In the UK, NHS guidelines recommended 700mg of calcium each day for adults, ideally from food sources. For midlife females this can be higher and for postmenopausal women it increases to 1,200mg per day. Be sure to check the recommended daily allowance for your age range and think about easy ways you can stay on top of this for your own sleep health.

- Pay attention to vitamin D as it helps to maintain a healthy circadian rhythm, support our immunity and maintain bone and muscle health (see page 119).

ACTION: UPGRADE YOUR RECOVERY HABITS

What has resonated with you so far in terms of the nutritional choices you can make?

- Is there a new daily choice you can make to support your sleep health?

- Have you had enough sleep-friendly foods, fibre and protein today?

HYDRATION AND SLEEP HEALTH

An increasing amount of research is exploring the links between hydration and sleep.[48] There are two sides to the hydration coin and, once again, it's all about balance: you need to be properly hydrated to enjoy great sleep quality and duration overnight, but you also don't want to drink too much too close to bedtime as it may wake you up in the early hours.

Frequent urination at night, known as nocturia, is a really common sleep hurdle. Nocturia can interrupt sleep with repeated trips to the bathroom and can be especially problematic for people who struggle to fall back asleep. In some cases, it may be unavoidable that you'll have to wake up at least once in the night to pee. This is normal for many people and becomes much more common during pregnancy, midlife and with some medical conditions or medications. It is especially prevalent in those who are over 60 years old.

If you frequently find yourself thirsty at night, it might mean that you aren't staying well hydrated during the day. Not only will dehydration affect your everyday life and health, but it will also impact your quality of sleep too. Even though your body is mostly still while you sleep, it's actually an active period when your body restores chemical balance, heals and recovers.

Dehydration can definitely have an impact on your sleep. If you are really dehydrated and lacking in certain minerals and electrolytes, perhaps after doing sport during the day, you may experience muscle cramps or restless legs, which can keep you awake. You may also feel tired and sluggish when you wake up the next day.

Your hydration level when you go to bed has a direct impact on the restfulness of your sleep. A hormone called vasopressin is secreted while we sleep to prevent dehydration by increasing the amount of absorption in the kidneys. This important hormone is responsible for keeping us from dehydrating when we go eight hours without a drink. When you're dehydrated in your sleep, you may experience excessive thirst in the mornings, headaches, dry mouth, muscle cramping and more.

Staying properly hydrated is so underrated for sleep health and, once again, it starts during the daytime.

ACTION: RESET YOUR HYDRATION RHYTHM

This week, focus on limiting any liquids in the final hour or two before bed. Make your choice, whether this includes water, herbal teas, alcohol or caffeine (which is also a diuretic). Consider the points below to help you embrace easy ways to do this:

- Sip, sip, sip: spread out regular hydration breaks throughout the day. An easy way is to add a glass of water to each and every loo or hot drink break.

- Reduce fluid consumption in the hour or two before bed. While it's fine to sip water, try not to take in large quantities of any drink in the lead-up to bedtime.

- If you consume alcohol, really pare it back to very early evening at the latest. Ideally, limit alcohol at night as, due to its diuretic effect, it makes you need to pee during the night and disrupts your sleep depth and duration.

For so many doing the Sleep Reset, these simple habit changes have had a huge impact on their sleep quality.

LATE-NIGHT SNACKING

A common nutrition trap I see with clients that can hinder wind-down and sleep is late-night snacking. Remember, sleep starts the moment you wake up, so how you eat during the day can have an impact on your behaviour in the evening, especially when you're tired.

When we're well slept and have a good mindset during the day, it's much easier to manage our food choices. Towards the end of the day, when we are tired, we are more prone to mindless – often sugar-filled – snacking. Very often when this happens we are meeting an emotional need and stress-eating rather than actually needing that snack.

If this is you, the 'Press Pause on Energy Stealers' mindset tool on page 139 will be the habit swap you need to stop this common sleep trap.

Lia approached me through their work sleep health scheme because they were struggling with sleep quality and duration. We started with laying the strong foundation of mindset, timing and light, but when we unpacked their daily nutrition they were really interested in looking at the impact of their hormones and the habit of constant 'healthy' grazing. Lia chose to spotlight the science of sleep-friendly nutrition. They were able to make some sleep-friendly choices across their day, increasing their protein intake and plant variety, as well as adding in more magnesium and fibre while balancing their hydration really well during the day. What was especially impactful was focusing on the evening meal to feature tryptophan-rich foods and swapping an early-evening energy drink for a caffeine-free sleep-friendly tea.

Lia really appreciated how their sleep health could easily be benefited by their daytime habits. This simple new focus helped them feel more energised and the realistic approach of a few small tweaks helped optimise their sleep and improve their focus.

STIMULANTS THAT DISTURB OUR SLEEP

Alcohol: why the nightcap disrupts your sleep

Alcohol is a sedative; it may fool you into falling asleep faster, but this is effectively 'junk food' sleep as it doesn't allow your body to benefit from the full restorative sleep cycles (see page 87), which means you won't feel rested and energised the next morning.

A 2021 study involving almost 12,000 people found that alcohol was associated with poor sleep quality, a greater likelihood of snoring and less time spent actually sleeping.[49]

Be mindful that your evening glass or two of wine or beer can block your access to good-quality sleep. Alcohol prevents you from entering the deeper, much-needed REM stage of sleep and makes you groggy and sluggish in the morning.

Caffeine: the real skinny on that afternoon caffeine hit

While it's true that some types of caffeine have natural antioxidants, when it comes to sleep, the picture is far from positive.

One of the things we know about caffeine is that it is rapidly absorbed by the body. Studies show that levels of alertness peak within 30 minutes of consuming it.[50] However, the half-life of caffeine – that is, the time it takes the body to eliminate 50 per cent of what was consumed – can be very different for different people. Research shows that the half-life of caffeine can last between two and ten hours.[51] Broadly, everyone metabolises caffeine a little differently, depending on their age, body weight, certain medications, liver health and sensitivity to caffeine. A general rule of thumb if you're serious about sleep health is to avoid all types of caffeine from mid-afternoon.

One study found that consuming caffeine six hours before bedtime reduced total sleep time by one hour. These effects can also be stronger in older adults aged between 65 and 70 as it takes their bodies longer to process caffeine.[52] It's therefore important to understand that all caffeine, in drinks and foods, has a very long alerting tail, long after you eat or drink it. Depending on your metabolism, if you were to have a cup of coffee at 1pm, a quarter of that cup may still be in your system at 10pm.

In sport, caffeine is a well-known and fast-acting performance aid within controlled conditions, and an effective agent for keeping you awake and alert. It can also have a positive effect on your reaction times, mood and mental performance because caffeine is a nervous system stimulant. On the flip side, it masks fatigue, and while it might trick you into a temporary boost of energy, it catches you out later as it steals your sleep quality, ultimately making your wind-down into sleep more challenging.

Indeed, new research is shining a light on the fact that our regular morning espresso or skinny latte might be delaying our body clocks and shifting our circadian rhythms.[53] Many studies have demonstrated the full effect caffeine has on the body clock and sleep health, with one particular study showing that caffeine inserts a slight delay in our circadian rhythm.[54] Essentially, this means that we nudge ourselves to not feel tired until later and later and get trapped in a vicious cycle.

THINK ABOUT THE SLEEP HEALTH CHOICES YOU WANT TO MAKE WHEN IT COMES TO CAFFEINE.

The way caffeine works on a molecular level is sneakily similar to adenosine, the natural chemical that our brain produces while we are awake that helps to create the pressure to sleep as it builds up throughout the day (see page 66 for a refresher on this). Caffeine targets the same brain receptors as adenosine, blocking its path. This is why we don't feel tired after drinking coffee initially and therefore may be tempted to stay up later and subsequently miss our sleepy bedtime cue.

THE WIND-DOWN NIGHTMARE OF CAFFEINE

Caffeine crushes sleep health in three sneaky ways:

1. It activates your nervous system and fuels anxious feelings. It also ramps up your heart rate.

2. The caffeine crash is very real. Caffeine is only ever a short-term fatigue mask.

3. Caffeine is so powerful that, in one study, one cup before bed (200mg) interfered with the stages of deep sleep - reducing them by 15-30 per cent![55] You wouldn't be aware of this the next day, other than feeling tired and unrefreshed, and will likely reach for another coffee shop hit.

A cup of coffee has an average of 95mg of caffeine – around double the amount of caffeine as a cup of black tea. Black tea is rich in antioxidants and recently published research suggests this natural flavonoid may mitigate the impact of sleep deprivation.[56]

Not a tea drinker? Not to worry – flavonoids are also found in lots of other food and drink, including apples, blueberries, oranges, dark chocolate and red wine.

Caffeine is also found naturally in dark chocolate. In fact, a 50g bar of high-quality dark chocolate contains around 25mg of caffeine. As a dark chocolate fan, this fact keeps me mindful to have only a square or two in the afternoon so it doesn't have a big impact on my sleep.

THE RISE OF CAFFEINATED FOODS

It's generally known that caffeine is found in dark chocolate, protein energy bars, cola and tea, but never before have so many processed foods containing caffeine been available. In one study over 4,500 processed foods containing caffeine were listed, and at least 262 brands of energy drinks are available globally.[57] From headache tablets to waffles, jelly beans to syrup, and even bottled water, the array of new caffeine-containing energy products seems to be ever-increasing. Look out for the words 'contains caffeine' when making your food and drink choices.

It's absolutely no problem if you love the ritual of having your cup of tea or coffee and it is purely for enjoyment. However, if it's costing you your sleep health later on, it might be worth a reset.

To avoid caffeine creating sleep turbulence, try setting a time boundary in your day, beyond which you won't drink coffee and will try to limit your intake of other forms of foods containing caffeine.

Try to forgo the habit of having a cup of coffee first thing in

Not all caffeine is created equal

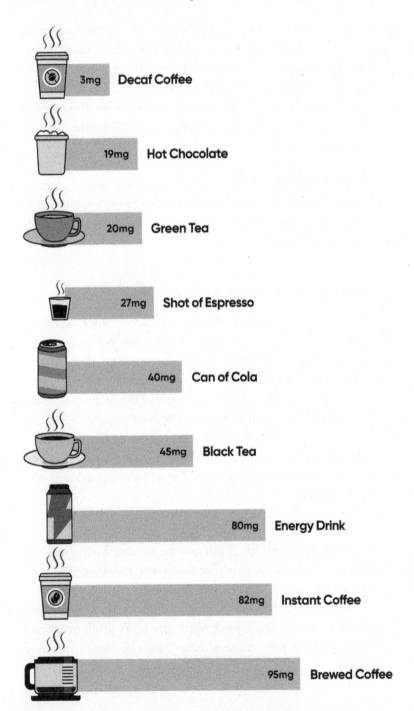

Decaf Coffee — 3mg

Hot Chocolate — 19mg

Green Tea — 20mg

Shot of Espresso — 27mg

Can of Cola — 40mg

Black Tea — 45mg

Energy Drink — 80mg

Instant Coffee — 82mg

Brewed Coffee — 95mg

the morning. Wait until you're fully awake and then have a great social cup in the mid-morning phase of your day.

I personally choose to enjoy coffee as a morning ritual and don't drink it after 2pm, but everybody is different. Try to be mindful about your caffeine intake, especially closer to bedtime. This book is all about focusing on you as a unique sleeper. If you enjoy drinking caffeine in the afternoon, this week you could try to bring it back one or two hours earlier and conduct your own sleep study. You may find it was just a habit that you can easily leave behind now that you understand its impact on feeling sleepy and your sleep quality.

THE LOW-DOWN ON DECAF

Very often there is still trace caffeine in decaffeinated products ('de' doesn't mean 'zero' caffeine; sometimes it just means a lot less) due to the process of production. However, it's still a great-tasting option when it comes to sleep, BUT not right before your wind-down. As ever, make the choices that are right for your current sleep health.

There is a growing market for high-quality sleepy teas – chamomile tea is one of the world's most popular teas for good reason. It has a phytonutrient content, specifically apigenin, which is proven to have sedative effects as well as reducing inflammation and oxidative stress and improving blood sugar regulation. A 2015 study focused on female sleep and championed chamomile tea as a natural intervention for depression and sleep disorders.[58]

Herbal teas that don't come from the *Camellia sinensis* plant (or tea plant) are caffeine free. This includes fruit teas, chamomile, ginger, peppermint and rooibos. Green tea, on the other hand, does naturally have some caffeine in it. However, while green tea gives you a small caffeine boost, it has tremendous wider health benefits and, in my view, tastes delicious.

Green tea also contains the amino acid L-theanine, which can cross the blood–brain barrier. It is particularly rich in polyphenols, which contribute additional antioxidant and anti-inflammatory properties, and green tea is exceptionally high in flavonoids, which are super beneficial for heart health.

Swapping to sipping green tea can be a really useful ritual for achieving a stable, energising curve with less impact on your sleep than black tea or coffee. I also find antioxidant-loaded matcha green tea gives me a smoother boost than coffee, creating alertness without the jittery effects.

ACTION: BREAK THE HABIT CHAIN

When I host sleep retreats at which people have a whole week away from caffeine, they are often surprised by how quickly they move past the caffeine habit and start sleeping longer. Understandably, when we reduce caffeine we can sometimes experience a caffeine 'hangover', such as headaches or generally feeling a bit rubbish. However, in my experience, the promise of better sleep quality makes it worth it in the end and, remember, you are fully supported with the audio tools to energise you in a more beneficial way.

This week, you can choose to move away from old habits and short-term crutches and finally invest in your long-term sleep health. To break the habit chain, you have three choices:

1. You could go all-in and give yourself a complete caffeine holiday. You might find that you never go back.

2. You could pare back your caffeine intake throughout the day.

3. You could focus on cutting back in the afternoon and evening only and swap to a sleep-friendly drink of your choice.

If your answer to option 1 is a resounding 'no way', consider the questions below when thinking about your own 'pick-me-up ritual' – it's worth considering what's driving this must-have caffeine habit:

- What does your MORNING tea or coffee really represent? Does it actually mask your poor quality sleep and act as a crutch? If so, can you swap to hot lemon, ginger or a turmeric tea instead?

- What does your AFTERNOON habit represent? If it is just a break or social ritual, can you perhaps choose to make a swap away from caffeinated drinks or high-sugar pick-me-ups to help your sleep health?

- What does your EVENING coffee represent? What could be a more useful bedtime drink for you? Maybe something warming without the caffeine?

Reviewing these questions should support you in making some sleep well-being choices and having self-awareness over your caffeine habits.

I don't want to nanny you here. As we've seen, tea and coffee have many health benefits, as well as bringing social connection. I simply want to support you in waking up to the sleep health choices in your hands each day and help guide you away from the autopilot habits that may be sabotaging good sleep well-being or masking poor sleep.

Remember this: your personal best sleep trumps any caffeine ten times over for giving great focus, sharpness and presence to your day. Sleep really is the great performance hack to your mind and body working 24/7.

CHRONO-NUTRITION: BODY CLOCK EATING

A good basic knowledge of the foods that protect or disrupt our sleep will help you reset in times of turbulence, but if dietary changes feel too much or are not possible due to financial stress, you can always think about creating a bigger gap between your evening meal and your bedtime.

Sleep is already your mind and body's natural fasting zone, but in the modern world we often snack or mindlessly eat across a big window of time from 7am to 9pm – or even later. Healthy sleep can be compromised by overeating, eating at the wrong times or eating too close to bedtime. This is also influenced by your chronotype – which you have already learned about in Week 2 – and whether you have a natural preference to consume food later in the day. As a strong 'lark', my body's preference is to eat earlier. Across 24 hours, even our blood sugar follows its own circadian rhythm, so it's important that we try to make better choices about how – and when – we eat.

Just as we have a sleep window, where we feel sleepy at night and alert in the morning, there is also a more beneficial eating window. You may have heard of time-restricted eating (TRE), pioneered by Dr Satchin Panda of the Salk Institute in California.[59] TRE is also known as 'chrono-nutrition' and is often practised by those who want to time their food intake with their body clocks. It is a daily eating pattern in which all nutrient intake occurs within a few hours (usually ≤12 hours) every day. TRE is about optimising the timing of meals for the benefit of our circadian rhythm and metabolic health.

Establishing an eating window of 8, 10 or 12 hours a day allows for a consistent resting fast to occur every day in the remaining 12–16 hours.

Chrono-nutrition is an emerging field of nutritional science that aims to develop an understanding of how when we eat can impact our health. This is an exciting area of behavioural sleep medicine and Professor Tim Spector at King's College London is leading some great research in this area.[60] When it comes to sleep, specific research has highlighted that TRE interventions prolong sleep duration.[61]

Fasting is an ancient tool that supports recovery and sleep and balances focus/energy. Sleep-related fasting is particularly important for repair functions in the gut, brain and liver. TRE may also be beneficial in the treatment of hypertension (high blood pressure) and managing healthy weight and stabilising blood sugar.[62]

ACTION: FLIP YOUR METABOLIC SWITCH

Could your eating pattern benefit from a regular and timed rhythm for sleep health? Generally, when I'm working with healthy adults, I help them choose a 'feeding window' that's right for them. Some people start with eating within a 10–12-hour window; for others, they are fascinated by the sleep benefits and choose to eat within a 6–8-hour window. Research highlights that it could be best to eat between 10am and 6pm.[63] This is something that I've found realistic and doable for me, but I'm not a slave to it if I have to travel extensively for work or am on holiday with my family. Make the choice that is most useful for your health right now.

I have witnessed so many clients struggling with late-night eating and poor sleep quality. When they flipped this simple metabolic switch they managed to see some really quick sleep health benefits from a ten-hour eating window each day. It can be as easy as that.

THE GUTSY STORY OF YOUR SLEEP

Your healthy gut is filled with unique, diverse combinations of bacteria. That microbiome changes when you regularly don't sleep enough. In simple terms, our sleep assists the smooth functioning of our digestive system through rest and repair; conversely, lack of sleep can have a negative impact on this.

In one study, researchers looked at samples of the participants' gut bacteria and sleep over a 30-day period.[64] They found that increased microbiome diversity correlated with longer sleep times and better sleep efficiency. The results also showed that specific types of bacteria (the trillions of bacteria and other microscopic organisms that live in your gut) were associated with increased sleep efficiency, while other types of bacteria were linked to measures of poorer sleep quality.

The range of 'good' and 'bad' microbes in your gut has been linked to how well you sleep, and some researchers believe that changing your microbiome can improve your sleep.

There is a fascinating interplay between the timing of our food, our gut health and our sleep well-being. The relationship between sleep and our gut microbiome – our internal microbial ecosystem – is likely to affect sleep and sleep-related physiological functions in a number of different ways: potentially shifting circadian rhythms, altering the body's sleep–wake cycle and affecting the hormones that regulate sleep and wakefulness.[65]

A 2019 study found that having a diverse microbiome – one with a wide range of different microbes – was linked to better quality sleep and a longer sleep time. It also showed that specific types of bacteria were associated with better sleep, while other types of bacteria were associated with worse sleep.[66]

New studies out of Japan suggest that the connection between gut health and the mind – known as the gut–brain axis – is so strong that it can actually impact our sleep each night.[67] Lead researcher Professor Masashi Yanagisawa of the University of Tsukuba explains, 'We found that microbe depletion eliminated serotonin in the gut, and we know that serotonin levels in the brain can affect sleep–wake cycles. Thus, changing which microbes are in the gut by altering diet has the potential to help those who have trouble sleeping.'[68]

Frustratingly, if we are short on sleep, this can mess with our gut health, increasing inflammation and stress hormones and altering our microbe community in as little as two nights, which might explain why not getting enough sleep is linked with worsening gut symptoms, especially for those with IBS or IBD.[69] Your gut bacteria have a circadian rhythm, just like the rest of your body, and get stressed out when you don't sleep.

It's clear that gut health/gastrointestinal complaints are

associated with sleep disruptions. People with insomnia report 20 per cent more gastrointestinal problems than those sleeping well and, conversely, people with gastrointestinal complaints report more sleep disturbances and, in some studies, as much as a 50% increase in chronic insomnia compared to the general population.[70]

Three (of many) ways that sleep deprivation affects our gut-brain digestive system:

- 1. Increases inflammation in the gut lining.

- 2. Increases blood sugar insulin sensitivity.

- 3. Causes hormonal disturbances that increase cravings.

Aim to make your meals more gut-friendly by eating a wide range of whole, fresh, unprocessed foods. A wide body of research points to the helpful effects of fermented foods for long-term sleep health. If you want to try this, include a variety of fibrous and fermented ingredients like kimchi, kombucha, sauerkraut and kefir, leafy green vegetables and probiotic yoghurt as well as nutrient-rich, health-boosting green tea, berries and sprouted seeds. However, I'm very mindful here of you supporting your personal gut health. My daughter, from birth, has struggled with childhood IBS and a highly sensitive gut. Very often, people with sensitive gut health need to take this journey slowly and also to seek nutritional guidance. I've learned this trial-and-error approach while supporting my daughter over the last decade. Now in her teens, we include a daily dose of kefir made from goat's milk because it contains tryptophan (see page 109) and live bacteria to support the gut. It's also a natural sleep aid of choice for me.

Achieving an 80/20 balance

Now that you are more aware of the impact of nutrition on sleep health, you can also enhance your sleep well-being by keeping some regular consistency in your patterns.

I often hear from clients about how changes in food timing over the weekend affect their sleep patterns and quality – and this comes as no surprise to me. Generally the weekend accounts for a big shift in behaviour: consumption of alcohol and caffeine increases for many and we reach for UPFs and go to bed much later. For many people when I start sleep coaching, they are missing out on five sleep cycles over what is essentially a three-day weekend. (Let's be honest, we tend to go on autopilot and change our habits from Friday breakfast through to Sunday night!)

There are no surprises when it comes to the list of sleep-trashing offenders that often dominate our intake at weekends. I expect most of you are aware of the obvious fact that late-night spicy food doesn't always equate with restful sleep. This is the same for caffeinated foods and beverages, added sugar, refined carbohydrates, high-fat foods and alcohol. There's plenty of evidence to link all of these to poor sleep.[71]

Of course, life needs spontaneous joy and social connections, so instead of an all-or-nothing way of thinking, or the perfectionist trap, could you reconsider your eating and sleeping rhythms to be more stable for 80 per cent of your time? Maybe on a Saturday you could then be flexible? Consider what works for you and is aligned with your Sleep Reset commitment (see page 36).

Habit change has to be easy, sustainable and realistic, but you would be really surprised at how quickly your energy, sleep and focus regulate when you don't have such a dramatic swing in your sleep and eating habits.

If I could prescribe a great sleep remedy, it would be to aim for a regular eating pattern within a window and a consistent wake-up time for at least 80 per cent of the week.

Aaron was a classic case I see so often of not making the connections between food, sleep and gut health. He had overlooked the link between sleep and nutrition and was propping up his low energy with unhelpful nutrition choices. The poor sleep and high caffeine consumption kept him further away from his health goals and didn't help him manage his blood sugar balance throughout the day.

He really appreciated the realistic 80/20 approach. We focused on supporting a TRE window for eating, creating a natural break from food in the evening; this was then an easy way for him to also stop the mindless snacking while looking at a screen he had been engaging in. He took a new interest in eating plenty of wholefoods and high-quality protein with a focus on adding colour and variety as opposed to food restriction and counting calories.

His daytime energy and focus expanded really quickly and his evening wind-down moved from solely sofa scrolling to a new mobility and power hour of self-care, starting from 10 minutes and effortlessly increasing to 30 minutes each and every evening. This was a strong recovery habit that felt essential as opposed to a chore or another thing he should be doing and he threaded it through every evening.

Many people I work with are unaware that their daily nutrition choices can also affect their sleep in positive – or negative – ways. Though I am not a nutritionist, I deeply understand the emerging sleep literature and I hope this week has helped you to recognise that your nutrition fuels good mental health as well as playing a supportive role in promoting your sleep health.

I hope you've found some new sleep-supporting nutrition tweaks that have sparked for you. However, if it feels too much for you or you don't have the capacity to make changes at this stage, at the very least it has allowed a recovery week for you to stay with what you have already achieved. Whatever pace you've been working to will be the right pace for you. It's okay if you have just stayed with the tools that are working well for you. You can always come back to this week when you have the capacity to look at your nutrition and hydration.

Next week, we'll be taking a close look at sleep stress and how you can overcome it.

WEEK 3 SLEEP RESET TOOLKIT

This week you've got a chance to review your progress, refresh any sleep routines and rituals and take a deeper dive into the links between sleep, food and mood.

Before we get started, and if you didn't do this when you first started the Reset, you can celebrate your new focus with a refresh of your sleeping space (see page 28) or plan a new well-being self-care ritual, such as a consistent digital curfew, a brand-new approach to your evening meal or finally ditching that sleep-stealing wine habit. Then look back at all you have absorbed this week and consider whether there are any tweaks you can make to your eating timing and habits. As ever, this book speaks to the choices you can realistically and easily make.

The tools this week are natural energy boosts and 'pick-me-ups' – there's no late-in-the-day caffeine required, no jitteriness and no subsequent fatigue crash. These are light-touch tools that are really easy wins to help fuel your sleep well-being in really practical and useful ways. They are all short but fast-acting ways to condition your focus towards your daytime eating habits. The good thing about the Sleep Reset is that you can layer in the tools in whatever way works for you. If things have been going well, it's great to keep up that momentum and keep your favourite tools from Weeks 1 and 2, while also adding in the new tools this week. Alternatively, you can simply focus on this week's recovery menu – the choice is yours, though try to carry on with the wake-up time and bedtime you set last week as best you can.

I wish I could sit down for a cuppa with you to help coach you one to one, but the tools this week have that tone in mind – I am here cheering you on the from the sidelines, whatever choice you make!

YOUR WEEK 3 TOOLKIT RECOVERY MENU

1. Your Mindset Tool: Press Pause on Energy Stealers (3-minute guided audio download)

2. Your Breathing Tool: Rest Espresso Break (3-minute guided audio download)

3. Your Sleep Hypnosis: Deep Body Relaxation Celebration Scan (30-minute guided audio download)

These tools are so easy and effortless, they will become as familiar to you as your tea break. This week, if practised, you can finally say that each day is peppered with rest and recovery.

Your Mindset Tool: Press Pause on Energy Stealers

This tool is super useful to help you with mindful eating and to notice how the food choices you can make are helping or hindering your progress.

This mindset tool will help you learn new ways to pause emotional eating and place yourself as someone who is really taking good care of your sleep.

The bonus here is that you also continue to practise calm, paced breathing control, which is so useful at night-time when you want to connect into relaxation mode.

I use this habit technique to help me keep a sleep health circle around my own TRE practice (see page 132), helping me have clear windows of mindful eating and keeping me away from mindless snacking. It acts like a habit circuit breaker, giving you more choice and freedom with snack habits you may want to set aside.

Your Breathing Tool: Rest Espresso Break

Inspired by my favourite compassion practice to teach (the classic Dr Neff self-compassion break), but here with my sleep health twist, this guided audio will help you to ease fatigue naturally and is a brilliant habit swap over not-so-meaningful scrolling. It will also energise you, instantly refreshing your mood and brain function and acting as a useful 'workday nap' strategy when a bed or cool, dark sleep space is far from sight.

I use this regularly as a useful daytime brain nap if I am on the go, and it turns out to be one of the Sleep Reset method's most loved audios!

We all experience that natural energy (circadian) dip in the afternoon and this tool helps you energise without the need for a nap or sleep-crushing late-in-the-day caffeine crutches.

Your Sleep Hypnosis: Deep Body Relaxation Celebration Scan

Planning and scheduling recovery is a great way to be intentional about your evening rituals and have a good sleep focus.

Don't skip this really powerful sleep hypnotherapy that makes lasting habit change easier for you, giving you space to align your sleep goals with the power of your brilliant mind. Deep down, this helps future-proof your new approach to sleep.

It also includes at the start a way to experience the mind–body relaxation of tapping and helps guide you on with good sleep breathing and visualisation.

Whenever you want to give your evening ritual a good boost you can layer in the sleep hypnotherapies throughout the book. However, this week, as it is chapter-themed, I suggest you stick with this one.

YOUR WEEK 3 BONUS TOOLS

Mindful eating mini exercise

A great tip is to power up your new-found breathwork and imagin-ation skills when you choose to eat. Here we create space and a more thoughtful approach to how and when you eat. A practical way to do this is to simply practise some box breathing (see page 49) or simple, connected breathing before you put food in your mouth. This tool comes into its own as you grow more naturally tired in the evening. This tool serves to support sleep in two ways:

1. It helps us step out of autopilot and consider whether what's on our plate is a help or a hindrance to our sleep.
2. It acts as a micropause to practise breathwork – in itself a moment of recovery.

Build a nap habit

If you have time for a physical nap during the day, instead of clos-ing your eyes, expecting sleep to come straightaway and being disappointed, download my 'Guided Nap' audio tool. This is great for those of you who normally fill ten minutes of naptime with Netflix or scrolling! This tool is pretty much the most valuable tool in my clinic and you can listen to it on a train commute or take that brain-boosting nap before 2pm to help manage the middle and later afternoon phase of your day.

YOUR REALISTIC SLEEP RESET 'PRESCRIPTION'

You've set some realistic goals for yourself over the last few weeks and practised the tools to get you where you need to be for your personal sleep health journey. This week you can take it at your own perfect pace – work with the energy you are building and put that good sleep quality into practical action.

This week, the ideal timing of the tools shifts focus to the middle and evening phase of your day – mid-afternoon and mid-evening. This is very often the time when we reach for UPFs that wreak havoc on our sleep well-being.

What is realistic for you to commit to this week – using these tools on two weekdays, four weekdays or just the weekend? As always, it's about choice.

Tool	Monday	Tuesday	Wednesday	Thursday	Friday	Saturday (optional)	Sunday
Mindset							
Breathing							
Sleep Hypnosis							

Hopefully by now you're getting more confident with planning your day, but remember you can always download a prescription for each week from my website: www.mindtonicsleep.com.

WEEK 4: COMBATING SLEEP STRESS

You achieved the energising midway point last week; now it's time to take another deep dive. This week builds on the skill of self-compassion, introduces you to gratitude and how it can anchor you into a sleep-friendly zone and furthers your breathwork with sleep breathing (slower breathing that promotes a relaxation response and helps you access higher-quality sleep). As you build on the Sleep Reset this week, you will learn how all these skills can help you when things inevitably get challenging and stress turns into a sleep-quality stealer.

UNDERSTANDING THE STRESS RESPONSE

Before we deep dive into the powerful effects of the nervous system in relation to sleep health, let's first explore what stress looks like in the body.

When we are faced with perceived danger or stressful situations, our brain activates the sympathetic nervous system, triggering what is known as the 'fight-or-flight' response. Alongside this, the hypothalamic pituitary adrenal (HPA) axis releases the stress hormones adrenaline and cortisol to prepare your body to fight off a threat or flee from a predator or enemy – your heart rate increases, your breathing becomes more rapid and your body tenses. The fight-or-flight response is an important aspect of our evolutionary inner system and is useful in certain situations, but when we are in this heightened stress response for long periods it can take a real toll on our health.

The mind-body connection

Our mind and body are in constant communication. It's hard to transition down into sleep at night when we are physiologically and biologically upregulated, with our foot on the gas. We're on, on, on, and our nervous system is flooded with stress signals and our sleep quality and duration are often impacted.

Left unchecked, this heightened stress response can fuel the HPA axis and mean that cortisol doesn't fade away as night approaches. Instead, it hangs around and can disrupt our sleep experience, both in pre-sleep and when we wake in the night and our minds race around at hyperspeed, quickening our heart rate and increasing our blood pressure.

COMMON CAUSES OF SLEEP STRESS

- unmanaged work anxiety and stress

- financial stress

- irregular bedtimes (aka 'social jet lag' - see page 91)

- unhealthy diet

- lack of exercise

- relationship problems

- trauma and grief

- chronic pain

- certain medications

All forms of physical and psychological stress can cause elevated cortisol levels and potential HPA axis dysfunction.

When we have reached our own unique stress tolerance, the stress system hijacks resources and tips our nervous system into hyper-arousal, where it feels like it is permanently switched on and on and on . . . whirring away in the background and activating the cortisol arousal system.

Research shows that heightened HPA axis activity is linked to more restless, fragmented sleep, less SWS (see page 85) and lower overall sleep amounts.[1] Research also shows that sleep deprivation and compromised sleep quality are linked to higher cortisol levels and to a more extreme cortisol response in the presence of stress.[2]

From a physiological point of view, you're in a stressed state because you're lacking sleep. On top of that, your thoughts recycle that stress. This loop is often referred to as 'the sleep, stress and anxiety cycle':

The sleep, stress and anxiety cycle

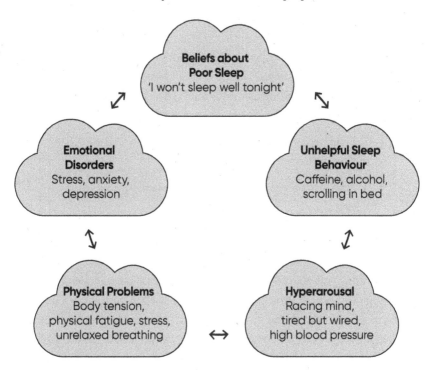

This everyday loop very often takes care of itself, but occasionally our stress perception increases and our body and mind send us the signals that we have reached our emotional load and sleep starts to feel stressed too. We accidentally become really good at elevating our own cortisol and thus shift the balance of our parasympathetic nervous system – commonly known as our 'rest and digest' system. In mind–body terms, this results in sleep, immunity and metabolic issues that show up as stress insomnia, tiredness, fatigue, brain fog and burnout.

> ADULTS WHO SLEEP FEWER THAN EIGHT HOURS A NIGHT REPORT HIGHER STRESS LEVELS THAN THOSE WHO SLEEP AT LEAST EIGHT HOURS A NIGHT.[3]

THE AUTONOMIC NERVOUS SYSTEM

This system regulates a variety of bodily processes that take place without conscious effort. This includes breathing, heart rate, sweating, digestion and much more. There are two branches of the autonomic nervous system:

- 1. Sympathetic: your body's ON switch, supporting mobilisation for action.

- 2. Parasympathetic: your body's OFF switch, supporting relaxation.

When we become out of balance with our stress response and everything gets alerted, the sleep stress loop is dysregulated and our energy sources are diverted. This results in sleep disruption or sleep that feels unrefreshing, and we start to get a sense that sleep is harder to come by – we experience challenges in falling asleep and being able to wind down, and struggle to get back into that relaxation response so crucial for sleep.

All day long your body senses the world and that information is transmitted through your central nervous system like a cycle route of communication. It makes sense, therefore, that if we have been distracted all day with tasks and avoided dealing with our stress, these natural arousal states and sensations can feel really 'loud' when our head hits the pillow at night.

Did you know that regularly having adequate sleep actually helps soothe the stress response and helps you process inevitable everyday stress? Very simply, when we manage stress, we sleep better, and when we look after our sleep, we can manage our daily stresses better.

ACTION: SET HELPFUL BEDTIME BOUNDARIES

A simple boundary I have is that after I brush my teeth at night I enter my recovery time. This clear boundary hour serves as a way to protect my pre-sleep relaxation and remind my busy brain that it is NO LONGER a time for planning, doing or work modes. Instead, this is the time for my creative mind - for reading or physical connection, self-care and self-love. I deliberately make no time for social media or doomscrolling and specifically make a habit of not listening to podcasts that are work-, health- or well-being-related as that is the theme of my whole day.

Be specific in your sleep commitment this week. Can you carve out your own recovery time - a new bedtime boundary for you that doesn't trigger work-related thoughts? Choose now something new to listen to or read that would soothe your daily stress and evoke relaxation. A 30-minute buffer before bed may be more realistic for you; that's still okay as long as you can try to consistently action it this week.

Aysha is a business executive who is dedicated and 'on it', enjoying life and taking health and fitness seriously. She has a jam-packed, 'optimised' day, consisting of back-to-back Zoom calls, meetings and deadlines while also squeezing in an hour or two of high-intensity exercise.

Aysha has a young family to care for so her high-tempo schedule runs from 6am to 10pm. Then it gets really wavy - she feels amped up and can't seem to wind down, with a racing mind and sleep anxiety. She distracts herself by surfing the internet, which only serves to wake her up more.

Her total sleep time averages five hours on a good night, but even if fatigued, she's up and at it again the next day, cracking on despite feeling time-poor and struggling to manage a high-pressure schedule.

Aysha's bedtime tale is one that may be familiar to you when life becomes too hectic. It is the perfect way to get 'sleep wrecked' – I hear it often from my clients. Our sleep can feel stolen by our mind and our reactions to daily stress and overwhelm.

Instead, there is another way. Learning to regulate your sleep stress and navigate sleep turbulence is achievable, regardless of what is keeping you up at night. It just requires a little commitment and consistency.

The times when you need a Sleep Reset the most are when you are lying awake with a racing mind, when you feel like you're waking up too early or are perhaps unrefreshed by sleep. You deserve to feel like you can make positive sleep health choices and get back to your best, most resilient self.

When we are stressed, our attention and focus get hijacked. Our motivation doesn't change; it is dimmed by mental events we label as stressful. Naturally, engaging in behaviour change sometimes feels harder.

The autopilot takes over and we stop being kind to ourselves and fall back into comfort habits and thinking loops that erode our sleep gains and give the microphone back to the rebellious, tired voice we saw in Week 1 (see page 47). We may fall back into a loop my GP friends have dubbed TATT – tired all the time – and feel self-defeated.

But you can dial down this sleep stress, triage when you need to and become much better at becoming sleep stress resilient:

- You can push that evening cortisol back where it belongs – far away from your sleep and only ready to help you in a good way to wake up.
- You can utilise self-compassion to manage stress perceptions in your mind.
- You can learn to modulate your stress response in the moment to help dial you down.

THE ONE THING WE HAVE IN COMMON IS THAT WE ALL EXPERIENCE STRESS, BUT WE ALSO ALL HAVE THE CAPACITY FOR CHANGE.

Let's start with unpacking the role of cortisol a little more.

The cortisol and melatonin balance

As we saw in Week 2, cortisol and melatonin are essential for us at the right times and have an important role to play in the sleep–wake cycle (see pages 64–70).[4]

Cortisol helps you wake up and is normally lowest around midnight and highest in the early morning, between 6 and 8am. Cortisol levels drop during the day, making way for the sleep-inducing hormone, melatonin, to help you fall and stay asleep at night. Problems occur when this gets out of balance or overstimulated.

Here's the part to remember: melatonin also operates within the HPA axis (the main stress response system – see page 143). So when something disrupts the HPA axis, it disrupts your sleep cycle as well. Increased cortisol suppresses melatonin and dilutes adenosine – the helpful sleep pressure molecule that helps you initiate sleep.

That's what is happening on the inside when your HPA axis is disrupted, but what do you end up feeling?

Just as we're settling in for some well-earned rest, we feel that familiar stress buzz and a racing mind and heart that seem so at odds with the resting body. In fact, left unchecked, this can turn into bedtime dread and start to fuel stress-related insomnia. If this is you, you might want to try the quick 'Stress Sigh Release' breathing exercise on page 176 to naturally reset and create instant calm.

Frustratingly, it seems that female sleep is even more sensitive to the effects of unmanaged cortisol. Prolonged high cortisol levels may change women's menstrual cycle because cortisol lowers oestrogen levels.[5] The result is a hormonal imbalance with symptoms similar to those of perimenopause: night sweats, sleep problems, mood swings and weight gain in the middle section of the body.

Sleep may also be worsened for women going through the perimenopause and menopause, because stress, depression and anxiety are known to increase during this time.[6] Levels of cortisol are higher at night-time during menopause, and they have been shown to spike just after a hot flush.[7] Both add to increased feelings of anxiety or alertness, often making sleep difficult. (See pages 247–254 for more on hormonal changes for women.)

But you can help prevent this night-time cortisol train from wrecking your precious wind-down and sleep well-being. The key is to level your cortisol naturally by finding ways to actively dial down stress and anxiety throughout the day.

The most effective way to do this is to get to know your magical inbuilt calm system: an aspect of your nervous system called the vagus nerve.

THE SECRET TO MANAGING THE SLEEP STRESS RESPONSE

The vagus nerve system acts to counterbalance the fight-or-flight system and can trigger a relaxation response in the body. The vagus nerve tells your brain and body 'you are safe' and is extremely beneficial for managing the real and imagined effects of stress and worry.

Simply put, the vagus nerve is the longest nerve of the autonomic nervous system (see page 152) and also happens to be one of the most important nerves in the body. It stretches all the way from your brain stem, through your neck, chest and abdominal organs to your pelvic floor and affects everything from your gut to your breathing during sleep. The vagus nerve is also closely associated with sleep quality. It balances the nervous system by promoting a relaxation response – a critical component of good sleep.

When it comes to understanding the vagus nerve and its calming impact on our sleep, you can focus on its role in one key area: the parasympathetic nervous system. Seventy-five per cent of this network of fibres, sometimes described as the body's 'rest and digest' system, are carried by the vagus nerve. Activation of the parasympathetic nervous system is required for quality sleep.

It's good to know that stimulating your vagus nerve could potentially reduce stress and lead to better sleep. A useful metaphor I share in my coaching sessions is that your vagus nerve is like a DJ, directing how fast or slow, loud or quiet your nervous system will be at any given time.

How to turn on your natural off switch

To help your body 'turn on' the vagus nerve to improve its function and help you soothe those stress signals, especially when your sleep is stressed, there are several social, physiological and physical 'tricks' that your body can employ.

One thing that's easy to do is cold water therapy, or placing

The Vagus Nerve: the Powerhouse of the Mind-Body Connection

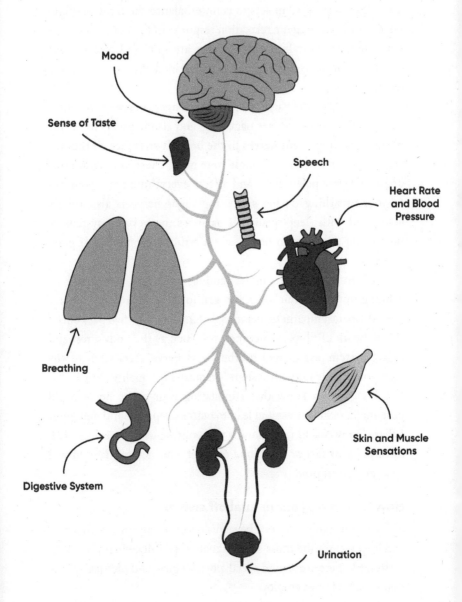

an ice pack wrapped in a thin cloth on your neck or chest. The research on this sleep hack is still very limited, but a small study from 2018 found that applying something cold to the outside of the neck can slow down the heart rate and increase vagal nerve activation.[8] Research has also shown that athletes experience a boost in relaxation after they immerse themselves in cold water.[9]

Below are five other ways to relax and stimulate the vagus nerve:

- Practising slow-paced breathing any time of the day will directly impact on states of relaxation or amped-up hyperarousal, which can steal your sleep potential. Slow, deep, diaphragmatic breathing that emphasises the elongation of exhales is key.
- Safely rubbing the inside of your ear (the bowl-shaped bits, not your ear canal), chewing food, sucking on food/objects and loud gargling all stimulate the vagus nerve.
- Massaging areas of the body that are linked to the vagus nerve helps provide a relaxation response. These include the muscles of the face, the side and front of the neck and head, the ribcage and the abdomen.
- Positioning the body in ways that compress and decompress the vagus nerve, such as rocking, which gently oscillates the head, neck stretches, abdominal and torso rotations, and gently flexing and extending the spine to affect pressure and/ or stretch. To me, this is a perfect encouragement for the bedtime stretching I advocate (see page 204).
- Meditation and some yoga poses, ideally with a side order of joy and laughter, also help activate the vagus nerve.

A COMPASSIONATE PATH TO OVERCOMING SLEEP STRESS

Working with stress-related insomnia or sleep challenges is really hard at times – it impacts on all areas of our day, leaving us feeling stuck in that cycle of sleep stress.

Learning sleep self-compassion is essential to help you:

- support yourself in a kind, friendly way
- not give up in frustration but find the capacity to keep going resiliently towards a meaningful goal
- protect your sleep health

I've seen how becoming compassionate is a very effective and useful mindset to finding a path towards better sleep health. When I was in Great Ormond Street Hospital with my son Jude, the ward had a unique feature: a beautiful sun terrace. It was a place of solace where I could ease my mind. At that moment, I found it hard to focus on gratitude so instead settled myself with short breathing exercises, such as 'Resting Down Overwhelm' (see page 172) that took me out of the stress response and into a kinder way to cope with the overwhelm (mindful self-compassion). In a nutshell, what I needed was an urgent mindset shift away from stress and into resilience. While the context might be different for you, the tools this week will help you do the same.

An essential part of improving your sleep health is understanding how self-compassion can help to significantly reduce stress day and night. Self-compassion is an innate capacity we all have in common; the ability to show kindness to other people can be reflected back to ourselves, especially when we face any sleep challenge. Self-compassion helps us shift focus from reacting to stress into a kind space where we can notice negative self-talk and take positive action for our sleep health and well-being.

As we explored in Week 1, when we initially face sleep struggles, instead of invoking self-compassion, we naturally tend to do the opposite – we aren't kind to ourselves. I like to think of self-compassion as the strength and conditioning to all areas of my work. Everyone can benefit from steady repetition and make gains from learning this valuable sleep health habit.

Let me ask you something: if a good friend told you that they have a new goal in mind, what would you say? Would you banter with them, sneering, laughing and telling them what to do? I bet you wouldn't reply with, 'Really? For real? It's never gonna happen, it's not possible – you will likely fail.' So why is it that so many of us speak to ourselves in this way when we are looking to prioritise our sleep health, especially at night, trash-talking ourselves and waking up to negative talk around our sleep?

A sleep-kind mindset will turn this habit around. At a time of insomnia and sleep stress, why wouldn't we choose to:

- give ourselves the same support we would give to a friend in the form of kind encouragement?
- forgive ourselves for perceived 'failure' and start again without any judgement?
- acknowledge that this is hard?

Self-compassion is essential for our sleep. We have to adopt a friendly attitude towards ourselves and understand when we fail or suffer, rather than trash-talking and ignoring our sleep health.

WE ARE NOT ALONE. IN THIS MOMENT,
PEOPLE EVERYWHERE ARE SUFFERING WITH
SLEEP AND INSOMNIA, AND THEY RESET AND
RECOVER. YOU CAN TOO.

I knew all of the above and yet, like you, time and time again, I didn't fully embrace self-compassion due to extreme fatigue and the mind and body stress of insomnia. It was easier to sigh, feel overwhelmed and keep pushing on with a playlist of self-doubt and stress whirring away quietly in the background.

In the midst of my toughest parenting and insomnia chapters came the breath of fresh air and knowledge I desperately needed when I discovered a revelatory book called *Self-Compassion* by Kristin Neff (see Resources, page 267), who is widely recognised as one of the world's leading experts on being kind to oneself. I started to explore the research and science of self-compassion that Kristin outlined and realised that this was a missing area of support that was essential for insomnia and sleep challenges.

Now is the chance for you to embrace self-compassion too.

Your self-compassion reset

You feel well rested, ready for sleep – and then your attention gets hijacked and you start thinking about work tasks, chores and conversations from the day, and that spiral that we saw in Week 1 begins. At this point you might ask yourself: 'How do I shut this off and clear my mind instantly?'

You already know that clearing your mind is impossible! We also know your attention is hijacked, so let's shift your mind to more useful places and guide it in deliberate self-compassion.

Think about how you can respond to tiredness in a useful way. Is your tone of voice friendly? When sleep is challenged, what will you choose to say to yourself that is deliberately kinder? Perhaps you can use an affirmation like: 'I trust in my ability to manage tomorrow with any sleep that comes my way.' It's essential you choose some kind of supportive chatter. If you don't, you can easily fall into the trap of a racing active mind once again or feeling stressed, worried or anxious. Every time you practise this positive self-talk, you mentally condition this positive rest into relaxation feeling.

ACTION: THE POWER OF AFFIRMATIONS

For most of my clients, at the top of their list is how to calm a busy, racing mind. I immediately share the science behind helpful bedtime self-talk, otherwise known as pre-sleep affirmations. Affirmations are a really powerful mind and sleep coaching recovery tool. Some really effective and simple deep sleep affirmations include:

- 'I am calm and peaceful now; I accept that my day is done.'

- 'My mind is calming down now as I settle to sleep.'

- 'I am breathing slowly and deeply ready for deep sleep.'

- 'I am grateful for this comforting stillness before my sleep time.'

- 'My mind is ready to be easily relaxed for deep sleep.'

- 'I am ready for rest and any sleep that can come my way.'

- 'Everything is just enough in this moment.'

- 'Letting go into sleepiness, relaxation takes over.'

It might feel counterintuitive to say something like 'I am calm' when you are anything but. However, repeating these affirmations consistently is a little like coaching a new reality that you want to achieve. I personally prefer a simple command cue to myself in a self-coaching style: 'Resting', 'Calming', 'Slowing down' or 'Ready for deepest sleep'.

I am curious; what affirmation would you choose?

Make a mental note or circle one of the phrases above so you can get on board with making this a habit.

Just try it every night this week and you will soon realise it's a helpful choice over the unfocused mental chatter that often runs away into sleep stress mode.

Instead of looking for a magic solution or a quick fix, the audio tools this week will further help you to develop the skills to move your focus in helpful ways and become more familiar with the recovery power of self-compassion. Self-compassion gives you a much more supportive, science-based alternative to close out your day to ruminating, rehashing your challenges and spiking stress.

THE POWER OF NATURE

When we get closer to nature in our day - be it the countryside, wilderness, beaches or woodlands - we really help dial back those stressors and in turn help manage our sleep well-being. Aside from the potent light benefits and positive effect on our mental well-being, viewing nature does our overstressed brains a favour. The gentle burbling of a brook or the sound of wind in the trees can physically change our mind and bodily systems, helping us to relax.

But what about at bedtime? Lots of people I work with are beginning to switch habits from bedtime scrolling to watching or listening to naturescapes as a way of winding down. And science shows that experiencing naturalistic environments (even through virtual reality, audio and video) can promote relaxation and well-being just like the present-moment experience.[10]

THE GRATITUDE BOOST

GRATITUDE
Noun. (grat.i.tude)

A POSITIVE STATE OF BEING. A FEELING OF THANKFULNESS AND APPRECIATION FOR SOMEONE OR SOMETHING; AND A SOCIAL EMOTION THAT SIGNALS OUR RECOGNITION FOR WHAT IS AROUND US.

Did you know that gratitude and sleep have a really cosy symbiotic relationship? In its simplest form, gratitude guides our focus to a 'state of thankfulness' for what we have experienced or already have in our lives.

Gratitude is positively correlated with more vitality, energy and enthusiasm. So many studies prove that practising bedtime gratitude can really help provoke a sense of safety and steadiness.[11] Gratitude is related to having more positive thoughts, and fewer unhelpfully ruminative, stressed or negative ones at bedtime. This, in turn, is associated with falling asleep faster and sleeping deeper and for longer. A night-time brain anchored with gratitude and kindness is more likely to sleep better and wake up feeling refreshed and energetic every morning.[12]

What I love about this science-based recovery tool is that gratitude immediately helps you focus on the power of the present moment rather than the past or future, without striving for constant achievement and change.

WOULDN'T IT BE NICE IF, AS YOU CLOSE YOUR EYES TO SLEEP, YOU ONLY CELEBRATED THE BEST OF YOUR DAY?

A common sleep hurdle when it comes to bedtime thoughts is that we have a negative bias towards the things we haven't done, haven't yet achieved or, crucially, the more difficult aspects of our day. A gratitude practice is a brilliant tool and skill to insert as part of your final wind-down. It helps you to lower any personal stress factors that can keep you from relaxing into sleep and conditions your night-time brain to shift focus to one good thing you can be proud of or celebrate today. Self-celebration is such a healthy way to wrap up the day and slow down thinking into a beneficial sleep well-being pathway.

Shifting your attention intentionally at night and choosing to focus on moments to be grateful for can improve sleep quality and lower states of arousal. This also has a really deep effect: at a neuro-biological level, gratitude helps us regulate the sympathetic (stress) aspects of our nervous system that activate our anxiety response that we have already learned so much about.[13]

Gratitude can boost the feel-good hormone serotonin and activate the brain stem to produce dopamine, the brain's pleasure chemical, which influences your mood and feelings of reward and motivation.

Practising the habit of bedtime gratitude has also been shown to:[14]

- help your brain well-being
- promote self-compassion and build resilience
- lower your blood pressure, useful for sleep
- improve your overall mental well-being and build a healthy mindset to help you deal with the inevitable stressors and challenges in life
- build some healthy adaptive acceptance in the face of challenges that we can't yet control

One study showed that over 40 per cent of individuals who suffered with a sleep disorder reported that they fell asleep faster and longer through practising regular pre-bed gratitude.[15]

Gratitude can be practised at any time, but a rest gratitude practice before bed is a potent tool to help calm anxious thoughts that can keep us tossing and turning at night.

Every night you will experience being alone with your brilliant but busy mind, noticing your thinking, reflecting on your day, your future and often feeling overwhelmed with all this 'pillow talk'. I know from experience that most people are not in the habit of self-celebration at the end of the day. Instead, the pillow talk is often when our stress, worries, unmet needs and anxieties come jumping up to the surface. Especially when our head hits the pillow and our eyes start to close, it can be easy to buy into the stress and unrelaxing nature of these pre-sleep thoughts.

We can proactively turn this around. A useful habit this week is to instead use this time to practise reflecting on and expressing gratitude for all the good – often small – things we overlook in our health and busy daily life. Helping your mind pivot from tasks and problem-solving provides a moment of rest to enhance your sleep well-being.

ACTION: **FIVE-TOE GRATITUDE**

A really nice habit I share with my clients that also helps shift from mind awareness into body awareness is 'five-toe gratitude'.

This body focus allows your sleeping brain to come home to your body and not stay up in your busy thinking mind. It will help you let go of that racing, planning mind habit.

Try it now – even sitting or lying down reading this, you can shift your attention focus (like a personal remote control) down to your toes.

As best you can, wiggle or move each toe on your chosen foot (it doesn't matter which) and match that with something that you're grateful for: 'I feel grateful for . . . in my day or this week' (remember, simple is always best). You can whisper it, say it in your head or speak it firmly out loud. Perhaps choose five people you are grateful to, or five personal aspects of yourself you are grateful for.

This is totally unique to you, but for ease I've included some examples for you to get going:

- 'I choose to celebrate this small win of my day.'

- 'Tonight, I choose to be grateful for my life as it is.'

- 'In this moment I will remember to express grateful feelings for my . . .'

- 'Right now I can focus being grateful on . . . no matter what.'

- 'I acknowledge I am grateful for _____.'

This action takes quite a lot of concentration – and with movement, thinking and body awareness combined, it's almost impossible to actively think of anything else at the same time!

When we start looking for things to be grateful for, we often find more as that focus expands and translates into well-being and stress reduction.

The impact gratitude has on the sleeping brain

Gratitude can have a surprising and powerful impact on your life by helping you to disrupt negative thought cycles and engage in positive mental patterns.[16] Research into how gratitude influences 'pre-sleep cognitions' (thoughts) suggests that by choosing to be grateful, people have more positive and fewer negative pre-sleep thoughts. This means focusing on calmer thinking that doesn't create the states of stressed thinking and breathing that make falling asleep challenging.[17]

Scientists conducted a sleep study in 2008 to measure the brain activity of people thinking and feeling gratitude. They found that gratitude causes synchronised activation in multiple brain

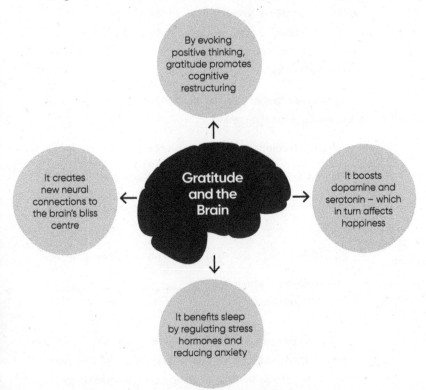

By evoking positive thinking, gratitude promotes cognitive restructuring

It creates new neural connections to the brain's bliss centre

Gratitude and the Brain

It boosts dopamine and serotonin – which in turn affects happiness

It benefits sleep by regulating stress hormones and reducing anxiety regions, lighting up parts of the brain's reward pathways and the hypothalamus and boosting our feel-good factor.[18]

When we express or receive gratitude, our brain releases a swig of mood-boosting dopamine and serotonin, helping us transition down more easily into restorative sleep.[19]

In one study, people keeping a gratitude journal slept on average 30 minutes more per night, woke up feeling more refreshed and had an easier time staying awake during the day compared to those who didn't practise gratitude.[20] Once you have embedded the five-toe gratitude practice into your pre-sleep ritual, why not take it one step further and keep a gratitude journal? What impact could this have on your sleep health?

ACTION: THE MAGIC OF JOURNALLING

Gratitude journals usually include a number of things or individuals you feel thankful for or moments that went well for you that day. Acknowledging the things you feel grateful for allows them to be more easily imprinted into your subconscious mind.

Once a day, in your rest time or as part of your wind-down, simply jot down three to five things from that day for which you're thankful.

Practising this gratitude habit every night helps you begin to reorient your pre-bed thoughts, focusing on more positive, restful things rather than just rehearsing the tough challenges of your day or what's ahead. I also find this easy to repeat upon waking, and it's certainly one to practise if you happen to wake too early.

Sleep gratitude helps widen our perspective and acknowledges the supportive connections in our day and life. Remember to switch your brain's natural negativity bias to positive feelings as you write your entries.

Acknowledging and appreciating what you are grateful for in a short and specific way soon becomes a bedtime habit that will immeasurably improve your sleep quality. If writing things down feels too much for you, you can compile a gratitude list in your head instead.

The breathwork practice and mindset audios this week will help you successfully build this gratitude habit strategy.

Michi, a third-year maths student, came to see me suffering from exam-related insomnia. She was particularly prone to a racing mind and giving energy to all the things that could go wrong in her week, especially as her head hit the pillow.

She loved the practicality of celebrating her day with gratitude rather than planning and worry. She was brand new to the power of sleep hypnosis and this week's audio tools became a comforting way to upgrade her bedtime away from mindless scrolling. The gratitude focus this week helped stop her tendency to ruminate last thing at night. Ultimately, self-compassion helped give Michi confidence in her sleep, and sleep care became her key priority.

Michi says: 'Learning the truth about my sleep health and training myself to be kinder about my sleep changed every-thing. These skills have helped me to build my confidence and understand it's essential to turn the power of my self-critic into my sleep self-coach. The sleep hypnosis audio this week really helped me to achieve this.'

EASY WAYS TO TAKE THE 'STRESS' OUT OF YOUR SLEEP SPACE

The impact of environmental noise surrounding us can have a surprising effect on our ability to wind down, our sleep habits and even our sleep across the night. You may like to consider some of the choices below that could be helpful for you:

- Noise-reducing earplugs: these can help you downregulate the nervous system and dial down sensory overload that may have built up during the day. We know we need to feel safe to sleep, so it's not practical to completely block out all noise. New affordable technology has meant an explosion in sound-diffusing earplugs. They don't block sound or make you feel isolated and can be safely worn as part of your wind-down and through the night. They reduce your stress response to annoying noises without blocking sound.

- Music: sound is one of the many sensory cues our brains tune into when we sleep. What we hear can have either a positive or negative impact on how we fall asleep and on the quality of rest we get. You may already be familiar with the white noise of a fan, but did you know that other soundscapes can have a beneficial effect on your sleep – from boosting serotonin levels to reinforcing a bedtime routine?[21]

- Nature sounds: did you know that sounds found in nature have a more soothing effect on us than artificial sounds?[22] Water sounds, such as rain, ocean waves or a babbling brook, are particularly conducive to sleep.

- Natural scents: this is an area I am passionate about. Natural scents such as lavender – which is the most studied and well-known sleep-supporting scent and itself a natural anxiolytic (an anxiety reducer) – help our nervous system to downregulate and prime the cue for the relaxation response.[23] Essential oils are really key here. Chamomile and jasmine are also particularly potent for relaxing the GABA pathways (see page 117), which is super useful for your inner sleep relaxation to begin. These two scents are a good alternative if you're not keen on the smell of lavender.

THE POWER OF SLEEP BREATHING

As we've explored, in prehistoric times, our fight-or-flight stress response was typically only activated short term in the presence of predators, enemies or other immediate dangers, but in today's world, the 'stress bear' is always there.

The sympathetic nervous system directs the body's rapid breathing response to perceived danger or stress situations. As we've seen, it can be useful at times, but is not something that we need to be switched on all the time, especially at night. The opposite number is our parasympathetic nervous system, commonly known as our rest-and-digest, sleep-calming inner system.

You can helpfully control these systems through resetting your breathing.

THINK OF TRAINING YOUR BREATH AS THE
WAY TO SELF-REGULATE YOUR SLEEP STRESS.

Low-level, constant daytime stressors tend to decondition us from our natural way of breathing. It goes unnoticed as most people are unaware of what dysfunctional breathing patterns are, but these will often result in tiredness, poor-quality sleep, stress and anxiety. Breathing re-education can help with dysfunctional breathing patterns and associated conditions such as anxiety, chronic stress burnout and sleep apnoea (see page 222).[24]

When our sleep feels wrecked, the best tool we can use is sleep (slow) breathing, which has an outsized effect on your sleep at night, not to mention your health in general. The efficacy of slow breathing techniques has been recognised by militaries across the world, which use such techniques during combat situations to regain composure and reduce stress.[25]

Regular practising of a slow breathing technique over time provides long-term correction of the hyperarousal stress response (sympathetic over arousal). In addition, slow, deep breathing has been shown to result in the production of the sleep hormone melatonin.[26]

As a performance mind coach and clinical hypnotherapist, I know that breathing helps to shift our state, enhances mind–body potential and harnesses incredible performance. You can think of sleep breathing as far more than just relaxation. You will have already felt the benefit of breathing exercises over the last three weeks. Now it's time to look at using breathing to specifically quell stress.

DIAL DOWN YOUR THINKING

Stress is a perception in your mind of a challenge, task or scenario that feels out of your control. We feel this stress effect in our thinking and in our body, but we can respond right here and now and start teaching ourselves to dial down.

A great way to diffuse non-stop problem-solving mode or self-defeating thoughts that prevent rest and our transition down into sleep is through the science-backed methods of sleep breathing and sleep hypnotherapy, teaching our deep subconscious mind that it's safe to get back into that soothe response. Deep breathing periodically helps to take your mind away from the 'what ifs' and the fatigued self-critical voice. This week's audio tools are designed to help put these useful skills in action for you (see page 171).

Many people don't make the connection between breathing and sleep. I learned the hard way during my twenties, when I sought help for an anxiety disorder. I'd have regular panic attacks at work. I was unaware of how to look after my mental well-being then, so it's no surprise I wasn't breathing in a helpful way. Very simply, I didn't have any knowledge or trust in the capacity for my breath to help me feel calm and in control. I wish I'd learned about breathing and the mind–body connection earlier. I can only imagine how much it could have helped my sleep and mental well-being.

We all experience disturbances in our breathing patterns.

The most common symptoms I see are breathlessness, stressed over breathing, panicky shallow breathing, light headedness and breathing anxiety at night or in the early hours.

Using your breath to hit the pause button and deactivate your stress

Slow-paced deep breathing exercises through the nose (nasal breathing) evoke a natural relaxation response. Slow-paced breathing is the best way to calm your nervous system, by initially slowing down and regulating a light, unhurried rhythm of breath, with your exhalation lasting slightly longer than your inhalation. This is the breathing technique that you will be practising this week with the 'Resting Down Overwhelm' tool (see page 172).

A recent pioneering study in the science publication *Nature* showed for the first time that slow-paced breathing is associated with increased stage 4 sleep – big, slow recovery waves that are associated with deep sleep, see page 87 – during the entire night, indicating that deeper sleep may be achieved with slow-paced breathing exercises.[27]

Slow, deep breathing has also been shown to result in melatonin production, which not only increases relaxation but is an essential sleep-inducing hormone as we learned in Week 2 (page 66). Reinstating the healthier slow and steady mode of breathing stimulates the body to spend more time in a rest-and-digest, restorative (parasympathetic) state. Sleep-supportive breathing – slow-paced deep breathing – also has a profound effect on all awake states.

Michael came to me via his GP. A hard-working husband and parent, his partner was diagnosed with Huntington's disease, which exerted extreme demands on his energy, crushing his naturally resilient mindset in the process. However, Michael was determined to thrive and do his absolute best for both his primary school age daughter and his beloved wife. The uncertainty of the future began to fragment his sleep quality, particularly as he had to be on high alert to respond to his wife's needs throughout the night and consequently had limited sleep opportunities.

We started by carving out a meaningful daytime practice that took just five minutes, using his breathing to regulate his stress and racing mind at night. Michael called this his stress 'circuit breaker'. For his part, Michael looked forward to creating respite in his mind through breath, which is portable and can be practised or invoked at any time, anywhere.

This meant he could weather this chapter of extreme pressure, protect his mental well-being and be present for his daughter, showing up with real value and integrity at a time of extreme sleep turbulence and trauma insomnia. Slowly, he was able to reclaim some great-quality sleep and achieve some much-needed rest and recovery. In turn, he could calm his thoughts and mind down into sleeping more soundly.

Slow-paced breathing not only helps with sleep stress but it can also improve performance and daytime focus, aid anxiety and depression, and help recovery from Long Covid and sleep apnoea (see pages 232 and 222).[28]

Another useful way to practise deep breathing is to reconnect with the three-minute 'Calming Box Energy Reset' tool from Week 1 (page 54). Box breathing, also referred to as square breathing, has four clear steps, just like the number of sides to a box. This practice can help promote equal breathing (where the inhale lasts

Deep breathing for sleep relaxation

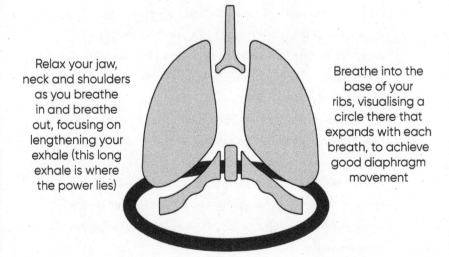

Relax your jaw, neck and shoulders as you breathe in and breathe out, focusing on lengthening your exhale (this long exhale is where the power lies)

Breathe into the base of your ribs, visualising a circle there that expands with each breath, to achieve good diaphragm movement

for the same amount of time as the exhale). Learning the art of paced, controlled breathing provides an anchor into the present, which aids the process of emotion recognition and regulation. It's good to remind yourself that breathing exercises for sleep don't demand much from us: we need only take deep breaths and, in some cases, count them out.

This week's focus helps coach you to strengthen your skills to shift down stress and enter your natural pathway into sleep, recruiting the friendly ally of your incredible vagus nerve and harnessing the science of breathing for good sleep quality.

Next week, in the last week of the Sleep Reset, we will look at the importance of rest and well-timed exercise to support and sustain your new-found sleep health.

WEEK 4 SLEEP RESET TOOLKIT

Over the last three weeks you have enhanced so many areas of your sleep. What often happens right about now is that your sleep is in better shape, and so the temptation to get back to busyness creeps in ... packed workday weeks, late nights and so on. However, the great news is that, by working on your Sleep Reset each week, you have already started to reprogram yourself to be sleep stress-proof, and I urge you to continue with the tools from the previous weeks that allow you to invest in your best rest strategies. However, this is the week when you can really start creating your unique Sleep Reset toolkit – for life. Layering this week's tool into your toolkit allows you to make a bigger leap into your recovery journey.

THE ACTIONS AND TOOLS THIS WEEK CAN BE USED TO HELP BRING TARGETED RELIEF FROM INSOMNIA OR AS A GENERAL BOOST TO YOUR WELL-BEING ALONGSIDE EVERYTHING YOU HAVE LEARNED IN THE PREVIOUS WEEKS.

CHOOSE HOW YOU RESPOND TO SLEEP STRESS

As we've seen throughout this week, sleep and stress are closely interconnected. When we fixate on a problem that is out of our control or a regret from the past, worry and rumination can take hold and further exacerbate stress and anxiety. By bringing our attention back to the present moment, tuning in to our senses and using our breath to slow our heart rate with this week's tools, we can deactivate our stress response.

We can never be stress-immune, but we can do our best to make ourselves sleep stress-proof.

If you are excited about the progress you've already made and the possibilities for looking after your sleep health that lie ahead, the themed tools this week help you address that ever-present stress sleep loop and help you take back some healthy control:

- Helping you navigate inevitable stress and, crucially, how you respond to it in more useful ways.
- Training the calming aspect of your nervous system to settle down that loop and get back to sleep when you need it.
- Getting to know your vagus nerve through this week's 'Resting Down Overwhelm' breathing tool.

YOUR WEEK 4 TOOLKIT RECOVERY MENU

1. Your Mindset Tool: The Gratitude Shower (3-minute guided audio download)

2. Your Breathing Tool: Resting Down Overwhelm (7-minute guided audio download)

3. Your Sleep Hypnosis: The Sleep Well-being Gratitude Scan (45-minute guided audio download)

This week's tools will help you embed a more helpful stress response that doesn't get in the way of your sleep at night and will dial up the sleep-supporting self-compassion, gratitude and breathing re-education skills you have just read about. The best thing about these deliberate practices is that they help you step out of autopilot thinking and recruit imagination, safety and care pathways inside, dialling down the stress response.

Your Mindset Tool: The Gratitude Shower

Now that you have learned about building a gratitude mindset, you can tap into the science of gratitude and its capacity to aid sleep with this guided audio that will help you tame any self-doubt/stressy thinking and instead offer you a science-based feel-good habit.

This is a well-loved insight that's helped hundreds of people. This tool acts as a healthy perspective boundary for me. It is like an invisible journal I take with me to sleep: I sometimes visualise it as a large blank page or a mental whiteboard – I have the pen and can write in a supportive way if I find myself in planning mode.

Your Breathing Tool: Resting Down Overwhelm

Welcome to this week's Sleep Reset breathing exercise, which focuses on slow-paced breathing and can be used at any time, but is particularly helpful in the early evening to combat worry. I also often do this after my journalling. This easy, focused routine can also be a calming transition/wind down right before bedtime.

Think of this as your very own resilience reset – helpfully shifting energy levels and finding clearer modes of thinking by tapping into your self-awareness.

These types of exercise elicit a relaxation response during which the body experiences a flood of calming hormones and physiological reactions that quieten the nervous system. Research studies have shown that breathing and relaxation exercises can help with insomnia, anxiety and sleep quality.[29]

The idea of this slow-paced nose-breathing exercise is to teach you how to guide yourself to reset your breathing down to an optimal six to eight breaths per minute. You might want to set a timer close by to gauge how you are doing!

- Step 1: Take a moment to settle into your posture, whether standing or sitting. There's no rush here, just notice how and where you are breathing in your body. Is it fast? Is it shallow?
- Step 2: Greet the breathing as it is and, after a count of five, gently guide it down into slow, deep, steady breaths as best you can until you reach six to eight breath cycles per minute.
- Step 3: Stay with the experience and enjoy the idea that each exhale energises your brain–body systems.

Regular practice will bring huge benefits!
This transcript is hosted on www.mindtonicsleep.com.

Sleep Hypnosis Tool: The Sleep Well-being Gratitude Scan

Now that your rest during the day is on the up, this week we can use your imagination to dial up your bedtime recovery rituals.

The wonderful effects of combined gratitude and sleep hypnosis are a potent way to continue looking after your sleep health. In scientific terms, meditation helps lower the heart rate by igniting the parasympathetic nervous system, or the part of the nervous system that helps you feel calm and regulated, and encouraging slower breathing, thereby increasing the prospect of a quality night's sleep.

Through this gratitude meditation, we can choose to focus on ourselves (our health, our talents, our energy for managing today and our feelings and achievements) and on our social circle (our family, friends and everyone else who unconditionally loves and supports us). This gratitude scan is an easy way to build your sleep self-belief.

You can practise this in the morning, any time during the day or as part of your wind-down ritual before going to sleep.

YOUR WEEK 4 BONUS TOOLS

Gratitude highlight reel

I wish I'd known during my worst insomnia that the gratitude mindset could lower my anxiety and support my sleep well-being. This is a simple, detailed memory recall exercise that can help you to build up the things you are grateful for and put them in your sleep bank. The positive effects can be felt instantly, making this tool an effective pre- and post-sleep well-being practice.

- First, focus on slow, deep breathing as you reach back in your mind to actively remember a time when someone was genuinely grateful and thanked you for something you did. Think of this as your 'gratitude received' story. Choose a personal experience or story that resonates with or is inspiring for you, one that you can easily recall.

- Think about how, with whom and where this gratitude story scene played out in as much detail as you can.
- Make some notes below, such as what the struggle was, how you were able to help and how it made you feel (you don't have to recall every detail perfectly).
- Now visually connect with it in your mind, repeatedly reflecting on this story, and gently breathe through this for a few minutes, really taking yourself there and recalling how it made you feel.
- Visualising this story every day will start to activate the positive parts of your brain. It's like the best mindfulness return on investment and helps connect us back with what is universally hard-wired – our capacity for storytelling.

_____

_____

_____

_____

_____

Replaying this familiar highlight reel has been proven to stimulate our helpful brain–body states, sparking your very own inbuilt gratitude system (super useful for pre- and post-sleep rituals).[30]

MAKE IT WORK FOR YOU

Recall your gratitude story and note it down on your phone or on a piece of paper as a cue to evoke it during the day - and rehearse the visual of it in your mind. Find something that works for you - perhaps a voice note will help you to anchor the story in your mind.

Switch position

A surprising habit twist if you realise your mind's active or you feel sleep stress tension/frustration rising just before sleep is to engage in a physiological mind hack. Very simply, switch position. For example, if you normally sleep on your side, try shifting over into an open recovery position, resting on your back. Very often, you will drift back down more easily. Everything changes when you switch position – your breathing opens, tension shifts and you are no longer stuck in a frustrated state. Try it tonight.

This is such a useful tool to have up your sleeve to shift that tired, wired, active mind and can also help you respond to wake-ups.

The stress sigh release

Learn how to find your focus quickly in a high-pressure environment using this anywhere, anytime, natural reset breathing exercise to create instant calm.

In order to calm down quickly in less than a minute, you need to make your exhales longer and more vigorous than your inhales. It's something we do subconsciously when we fall asleep – and even when we cry – so it's a great practice for night-time.

One of my favourite papers published in the *Journal of Neuroscience* demonstrates that the rhythm of breathing affects memory and fear and that there is a dramatic difference in brain activity in the amygdala and hippocampus (the centre of emotion and memory) during inhalation compared with exhalation.[31] In other words, when we breathe better, our mind helps our performance in many ways. Our inhalation amps us up while our exhalation helps to calm us down. This is why making our exhalation longer than our inhale is a fast-track way to bring calm focus to our brain and body.

This focused release exhale helps to activate the vagus nerve, which is connected to your parasympathetic system. Did you know that it is also connected to your vocal cords and the muscles at the back of your throat? This is why deep, long exhalations trigger it to work.

Think of this tool as your Sleep Reset secret weapon, super useful for panic and anxiety and fleeting moments of overwhelm, which are often especially loud at night, and perfect for those cortisol rollercoaster moments or to calm a racing mind, racing heart or stressed, tight chest. I love to teach this in all settings – whether someone is about to give a talk, on the pitch ready to perform or winding down last thing at night. Often during these moments we'll try to use the mind to calm the mind; in this exercise, we are going to do something strictly mechanical by breathing in a specific pattern.

This technique calms the fight-or-flight response, allowing us to regain control. Here's how it works:

- Take two rapid inhales through the nose, followed by a long, extended exhale through the mouth. Try to do the inhales through the nose, even if you feel a little congested. If your nose is totally blocked, breathe in through your mouth with pursed lips.
- Repeat this ten times, before returning to your normal breathing pattern. This is a brilliant, middle-of-the-night, sleep-soothing SOS tool.

YOUR REALISTIC SLEEP RESET 'PRESCRIPTION'

Now you're in Week 4, you can really think about using the tools across the span of your day, from wake-up to bedtime. Remember, you get to set your own pace and rhythm. If you can only fit one thing in this week, prioritise the longer sleep hypnosis three or four nights per week as part of your evening wind-down, or you can absorb this audio as part of an evening walk, where it will be working on your unconscious mind in the background, not putting you to sleep in that moment.

I challenge you to see how many times you can do the 'Stress Sigh Release' on your busiest day!

Tool	Monday	Tuesday	Wednesday	Thursday	Friday	Saturday (optional)	Sunday
Mindset							
Breathing							
Sleep Hypnosis							

WEEK 5: THE IMPORTANCE OF REGULAR REST AND WELL-TIMED EXERCISE FOR SLEEP HEALTH

Before we get started with this last week of the Sleep Reset, I'd like you to take a moment to think about all that you have achieved so far. You've made your own sleep commitment (page 36). You'll hopefully have discovered tools that work for you and have already integrated them into your everyday so that they feel effortless – and you won't now leave them behind. You also know how to troubleshoot and look after your sleep. There is so much value in the journey you've taken to make new choices and kick some habits out of bed – for good – and you can self-celebrate all of the tiny wins that will sustain your healthy new approach to sleep.

Don't worry if things aren't quite where you want them to be just yet or you haven't found the perfect time to implement all the tools. Just by reading this book, you are armed with the many ways in which you can choose to rest, recover and look after your sleep at any stage. If I was by your side, I would point out all the small steps of sleep self-care that are now embedded into your knowledge.

It's now time to explore how rest and well-timed exercise can deepen and strengthen sleep in equal measure, helping you to unlock your sleep personal best, fall asleep more quickly and improve sleep quality. Along with everything else you have learned so far, this really is the icing on the cake.

WHY REST IS SO IMPORTANT

JUST AS WE ARE ALL ADEPT AT GOING FROM 0 TO 100MPH IN OUR DAY, IT'S ALSO USEFUL TO LEARN HOW TO GO FROM 100 TO 0MPH.

Most of us have a PhD in busyness and yet not many of us would say that we're brilliant at rest. Rest is often overlooked, especially in the first few phases of our action-oriented, task-driven days. We need to coach ourselves to become as familiar with being still as we are with being busy.

As we explored last week, there are so many demands on our time – many of us combine jobs with caring and supporting multi-generational families, and then there are the never-ending tasks and errands of adult life. As we try to fit everything in, we often forgo our boundaries, staying up late trying to hustle our way through, accidentally sacrificing regular rest and sleep – and, some-what worryingly, this is a process that we repeat.

Every day, I see this negative pattern leading to outsized cause and effect. The switched-on, upregulated stress that we explored in Week 4 makes us forget that we have an inbuilt capacity to relax. It also erodes our mental and physical health. Undervalued and over-looked, the fact remains that sleep and rest – in other words, real everyday recovery – is absolutely vital to our well-being.

Don't forget that you were born with the skill to settle yourself and take a moment of rest. It's totally unique to you, but I under-stand why we all need reminding of how we can move into a rest moment.

What I see in my work with supporting high achievers and elite athletes is that their sleep is getting wrecked more often than not due to a lack of focus on deliberate rest, inconsistent sleep times and not taking steps to manage stress.

Over the course of this week we will discover why making the choice to practise deliberate rest in your waking state will help your sleep health and emotional well-being through the power of neuroplasticity (see page 46). Your goal is to learn how to make deliberate rest and recovery something you can call on whenever you need it – a tangible, built-in part of your day.

Learning to rest matters for your sleep health. Training yourself to regularly pause for a moment is essential to being human and to your own performance well-being. Alex Soojung-Kim Pang, author of *Rest* (see Resources, page 266), is one of the most influential voices on this subject. He helped to shape the global movement towards a four-day week and his book advocates treating work and rest as equals:

> 'You cannot work well without resting well. Some of history's most creative people, people whose achievements in art and science and literature are legendary, took rest very seriously. They found that in order to realise their ambitions, to do the kind of work they wanted to, they needed rest.
>
> 'Work and rest aren't opposites like black and white or good and evil; they're more like different points on life's wave. You can't have a crest without a trough. You can't have the highs without the lows. Neither can exist without the other.'

We touched on the impact of blue light and technology on our sleep health in Week 2. But our attention-grabbing digital world has further repercussions for our sleep – we do not value rest any more. Cast your mind back ten or fifteen years: what did your weeknight chill-out look like? I imagine it wasn't watching a big screen while also scrolling on a smaller screen, chin down and hunched over. In many households, 'rest' has evolved to be multi-screen-based, and this is secretly stealing our sleep opportunity.

This week will help you change that.

REST HELPS US SUSTAIN THE SLEEP SWEET SPOT.

Discover your own definition of rest

Deliberate rest is not just 'being', sitting inactive or lying around doing nothing. The kind of rest that leads to recovery, which we need for healthy sleep, is anything but simple downtime. It replenishes the brain, increases alertness and helps to decrease stress and feelings of overwhelm and fatigue.

> REST AND RECOVERY ARE ESSENTIAL – NOT JUST A 'NICE TO HAVE' ASPIRATIONAL BIT OF SELF-CARE.

Rest is any activity that allows our stress responses to 'switch off', activates the parasympathetic nervous system (see page 146) and shifts our body out of a state of fight or flight and into a state of rest and recovery. It is about entering activating states of relaxation, cognitive rest, attention refresh, stress reduction or body rest, and it can be really energising.

Depending on our beliefs and environment, our perception of rest can look and feel really different. Rest could be taking a deliberate moment to listen to one of the Reset tools, actively taking your lunch break, reading a book, going for a walk, connecting with somebody face to face or, very powerfully, considering how you 'unplug'. Redefining rest as unplugging is really useful because, for many of the people I work with, rest has become synonymous with scrolling or watching junk TV. When you swap the word 'rest' for 'unplug' it immediately opens up more imaginative rest possibilities.

Small defined pockets of deliberate rest give you more helpful control over habits and choices, keep you away from overwhelm and burnout, and help you maintain a healthy energy balance. Rest needs to be flexed every day for sleep well-being as it is what allows our minds and bodies to recover from the stresses of daily life so we feel and perform at our best.

> DO LESS AND YOU WILL ACCOMPLISH MORE.

I bet you already know that every day you practise ignoring your inbuilt rest signals. This is in no way a judgement – our modern world is designed to nudge us to do exactly this. It's common knowledge that our 'pocket' technology is designed to 'hypnotise' us to keep scrolling and clicking, and distracts us from feelings of natural sleepiness. It's easy to see how this has become an everyday sleep-time problem.

The hustle culture of the last 30 years or so has hidden a sleep health epidemic that is now really beginning to emerge. It's cost us our sleep and mental health and pressurised our mental well-being. That is why it's so normal to find it hard to find the time for rest and why your nervous system – which, as we saw in Week 4, is so used to being amped up all day and drenched in blue light at night – finds the stillness of hitting the pillow really hard at times. Without balancing the stress in our lives with rest, we build something called 'allostatic load' – wear and tear on the body caused by elevated hormonal and neural responses to stress.

Tricia Hersey, founder of The Nap Ministry and author of the *New York Times* bestselling book *Rest Is Resistance* (see Resources, page 266), makes a powerful case against hustle culture: 'This is a paradigm shift; it's an ethos that looks at slowing down and pushing back against a system that says our worth is connected to how much we've done.' I absolutely agree with her pushback.

ACTION: **WHAT REST MEANS FOR YOU**

Ask yourself the following questions. In your answers lies opportunity.

- What types of rest practices do you make time for on a regular basis already? Note how this potentially looks different in your workday versus your weekend versus when on holiday.

- Can you identify one simple restful practice that you could do every day, no matter what? A good example is to read just a few pages of a book every day or do a pre-bed restful stretch.

- What are the signs that you need to prioritise rest in your mind and body? This might look like neck tension, eye strain, feelings of overwhelm or feeling stiff in your body.

- What are the time barriers that can get in the way of getting enough rest?

- What might be some of the boundaries you need to set so you can honour your need for rest?

- Will you schedule rest more now?

Learning deliberate rest matters for your sleep health. Training yourself to regularly pause for a moment is essential to being human, to your own performance well-being and to reducing stress.

YOUR SLEEP IS YOUR BEST ASSET, NO MATTER WHAT YOUR DAYTIME LOOKS LIKE.

To get started with well-timed rest, there are a number of easy ways that you can incorporate it into your working day. The first step is recognising that cognitive fatigue is real and valid. Don't allow yourself to feel like a failure for struggling or think you can just 'power through'. You can't.

THE IMPACT OF COGNITIVE FATIGUE

Cognitive fatigue is a unique kind of fatigue or tiredness, or, as Daniel Goleman described, 'When our daytime brain gets too tightly focused, attention gets fatigued – much like an overworked muscle.'[1]

Mental or cognitive fatigue can be defined as a decrease in

cognitive resources (your brain's energy and focus) the longer your day progresses, especially when we spend lots of time without breaks or rest.

It is now widely accepted that 'thinking hard really is tiring for your brain' (beautifully outlined in a study that links mental fatigue to changes in brain metabolism).[2] People who spent six hours working on a tedious and mentally taxing assignment had higher levels of glutamate – an important signalling molecule in the brain. Too much glutamate can disrupt brain function, but a rest period could allow the brain to restore proper regulation of the molecule.

Cognitive fatigue happens to us all without our awareness when we have a number of demands on our thinking that build up across our working day. Even outside pockets of intense screen time, think of life admin: having to remember plans, WhatsApp groups, endless Slack messages, appointments, emails, notifications. These sometimes don't feel like cognitive fatigue or 'hard mental work', but they add up and take their toll.

It seems there is no escaping this build-up, but, once again, we can react to it in beneficial ways for sleep well-being.

SIGNS YOU'RE EXPERIENCING COGNITIVE FATIGUE

- You find it difficult to concentrate.

- You're forgetful.

- You're easily irritated.

- Tasks that should be simple feel difficult.

- You feel overwhelmed.

- You're struggling with sleep.

- You have physical symptoms of stress such as headaches, tension and an increased heart rate.

- You feel disconnected from the world, like you're in a dream or in a fog.

- You experience a 'mental block' - when you simply can't do any thinking.

It's really helpful to have small 'recovery zones' throughout our day. The 'recovery zone' is a simple, easy way to describe the natural zones in our every day when we have the capacity to choose to rest and work with our rhythm, not against it. I know that if I called this 'quiet time', 'self-reflection time', 'chill-out time' or 'slow moments', you might be tempted to skip this section!

Rest is not just nice to have to help us take a breather, it is essential for sleep health. When we look at balancing our nervous system, rest is so influential on our ability to sleep well. Remember the phases of the day we explored on page 90? There is a natural, 'hard-wired' fatigue slow-down in energy levels directly timed and linked to our circadian rhythm. This natural ebb and flow in our ability to feel alert or sleepy happens throughout our day, but in this attention-grabbing, brightly lit, noisy digital world we often miss these biological cues. We need to work with the natural plateaus – the dips.

We are used to overriding these small nudges to rest, which get drowned out by our light- and screen-filled worlds, but your brain needs some well-timed rest breaks to restore focus and composure. A simple hack for combating evening cognitive and eye fatigue is to consider some blue-light-blocking glasses to ease the strain and protect your sleep health (see Resources, page 268).

UNLOCKING THE POWER OF REST

SO MUCH TENSION IN MY LIFE EASED WHEN I
REALISED THAT THE BIG SHIFTS I NEEDED

ONLY HAPPENED BECAUSE OF THE SMALL
RIPPLES OF REST I HAD SET IN MOTION
EVERY DAY.

Daytime rest, which I define as real recovery, is a skill we deserve to develop and we should start thinking of it in that way. Not many of us would skip the opportunity to replenish our brain power, and yet we often choose not to rest during the daytime, missing out on an instant brain boost and the chance to protect our thinking and creative capacities. Sometimes, when I'm busy, I need to remind myself that daytime rest actually makes me smarter and my focus sharper.

If you want to strengthen your emotional well-being and sleep health, using these rest skills during the day is when the crucial change will happen. Through my work with elite athletes, I've seen this first hand in a sporting context, but it has broader applications too; we are all trying to achieve amazing physical feats in our own worlds every day. If you find yourself thinking: *No, that's not me*, hear me out. I know you will have great expectations of yourself, wanting to achieve high levels of focus for the tasks you have to complete each day. You deserve to enjoy meeting your own personal bests in life. However, you will need to build in recovery, just like an athlete does.

I treat everyone as an athlete, from carers who need the energy and resources to turn up to a challenging day at work, week in and week out, to frazzled parents struggling to contend with sleep disruption caused by their newborn baby or sleep-challenged teenager.

We all have natural, variable cycles of energy and pressure across our weeks and months. Just like the athletes I work with, we also have seasons of growth, rest and recovery, reflection and full focus.

We don't discover rest – we have to plan it. I'd like you to think about all the moments in the day when you have a few minutes to tap into confident relaxation. By doing so, you can access the resilience, creativity and clear-thinking moments that are often referred to as being 'in the flow'. Below are some helpful pointers on nine types of daytime rest:

1. Intentional time away: taking yourself out of your habitual routine and environment.
2. Permission not to be helpful: using self-compassion to practise the art of saying no and protecting your deliberate rest and sleep well-being.
3. Tech-free 'unproductive' time: allowing your scrolling eyes and fingers to step away from tech as you choose to do something for yourself.
4. Connection to art and nature: resting in nature has hugely positive effects on your health (see page 32). Your brain circuits react positively to the calming effects of surrounding scenery and environment.
5. Solitude to recharge: taking even one minute for ourselves alone allows us to step into the slow, deep breathing that brings real benefits.
6. A break from responsibility: when we're caring for others or doing our job, taking deliberate rest helps us become more engaged and alert, becoming the recharge we need.
7. Stillness to decompress: in stillness, we naturally close our eyes; choosing to rest them initiates a natural relaxation response.
8. Safe space: this is an opportunity to recall natural scenery that speaks to you, or instead you can use the 'Gratitude Highlight Reel' on page 174 to remember your gratitude story.
9. Alone time at home: you can achieve this by choosing to rest in your own particular peaceful sleeping environment or bedroom.

TRY TO BUILD A MICRO REST INTO YOUR TEA OR LUNCH BREAK SO IT BECOMES A HABIT.

ACTION: RESETTING YOUR APPROACH TO REST

Stop for a moment. When was the last time you truly relaxed? When was the last time you felt properly connected to the reasons for slowing down and engaged in recovery, knowing that it was an essential part of your daytime?

These days, when most people take a break, they are still screen-led, searching for more news, updates and visuals. Using the list above, take some time to write down your unique way to schedule just three minutes of deliberate rest each day - a sort of personal weekday rest recovery manifesto. Draw out some simple ways you can reach for recovery moments, even on those really busy, low-energy days, to take all the pressure off your racing mind. The key to building this habit is to make it easy, time-led and to enhance a natural break you already have. Three minutes of deliberate rest either side of your main meals each day is a great place to start. It really can be that simple.

Focus on the one thing you will do when things get really busy - this is when recovery is even more essential to diffuse mind and body stress.

You really don't need to wait until you are exhausted, ill or on holiday to rest. Recovery is an essential antidote to everyday stress and really helps you build up your energy bank and get your sleep–wake cycle back in a healthy balance.

ENVISION REST AS SMALL BUT CRUCIAL MOMENTS TO TAP INTO THE POWER OF THE MIND AND CHANGE YOUR BREATHING.

Embracing pockets of rest is a vital step in overcoming stress and anxiety and one of the core steps to building your sleep health for life.

GET OUT INTO GREEN SPACES

Green space is considered a critical environmental factor for sleep quality and quantity. Access to nature has also been found to improve sleep and reduce stress, increase happiness and reduce negative emotions.[3] If you can, try to spend time visiting natural places – green spaces like parks, gardens or forests, or blue spaces like the beach, rivers and wetlands. Try leaving the headphones at home – unless you're listening to nature sounds of course! Or why not try a new route to work or your kid's school that brings you closer to green spaces or water?

I love the emerging science that proves being out in nature in motion actually has physiological effects inside. When we walk instead of looking at a screen, our eyes switch to a wider focus – our very own panoramic vision. This is associated with improvements in both sleep quality and quantity.[4] Other studies suggest exercise outdoors and therapeutic gardening as possible intervention methods to improve sleep outcomes.[5] That has to be better than cricked-neck scrolling – looking down at small screens on our 'restful' lunchbreak – surely. This is a choice you can make.

Even in cities where nature can be harder to find, there are community gardens, courtyards or parks to discover and explore. Look out for the unexpected. Try to notice nature wherever you are, in whatever way is meaningful for you.

Just as there are green spaces for rest, we should also try to build more 'white space' into our working day. Adrienne Herbert, host of the wildly successful podcast and book *Power Hour*, has coined this concept. White space is time in your schedule for creative rest. As Adrienne herself puts it:

'We give our time, energy and attention to so many external things from the minute we wake up to the minute we go to bed. I think we have to be intentional about how we spend our time. We need to reclaim it, which literally means taking back something that was previously yours. Remember that your time is yours before you give it away.

'It isn't about more, more, more. It's not about the hustle culture. It's not about the perfect routine. It's about finding time for yourself before you have given yourself to others. And when you prioritise yourself in the morning, it is easier to carry on doing that throughout the day. It sets up your direction and your attitude going forward. The morning also feels powerful because you are so often without distraction.'

Create a golden hour for rest

For many of the tired people I work with, I prescribe a golden hour in the morning as a lovely way to focus on the art of complete intentional rest. If a whole hour doesn't feel achievable on a week-day, you can take this concept of a golden hour for rest and translate it to a golden boundary of, say, five or ten minutes each morning, and look forward to the golden hour ritual at the weekend or on a day that suits you instead. Again, it comes down to making choices that are beneficial for you.

I love this concept and I've become very intentional about how I use that time. For me, I don't want to fill it with life admin or add an extra hour of cognitive load. Instead, I use the golden hour to be proactive about my well-being goals: tuning into how I feel, doing some journalling or thinking about seasonal travel, places and spaces I would like to go. Planning in this way can feel restful and creative, not another busy task.

Finding a golden hour for rest in the morning very often works best away from interruptions and distractions. We all know that later on in the day it can be hard to cultivate that precious solitude.

Can you start this week with just ten minutes, or go for the full hour? How can you ring-fence this time in your diary? Perhaps look at your morning routine: are you wasting time scrolling on tech? Try to be more intentional and really home in on a slow morning. Or find an hour of calm focus: focus on one bigger personal project that's completely separate from your work and everyday life.

Overcome the guilt

Consider how loaded with guilt rest is sometimes. When you take time out for yourself, it provides you with a natural reset and it is incredibly important that you schedule, prioritise and protect this deliberate rest and recovery without guilt. As you learned in Week 4, self-compassion is a great way to jump over any past guilt hurdles or anxieties.

By now, you understand the importance of reframing your self-awareness and self-talk – in other words, your mindset approach towards deliberate rest. So step away from any 'learned' guilt about daily rest and recovery.

Unhelpful sleep mindsets we can easily challenge include:

- 'I need to earn rest.'
- 'I don't deserve rest, I have to push on.'
- 'Hustle and grind; sleep is something I can miss in pursuit of my goals.'

Some easy hacks are:

- Practise rest habitually three days a week.
- Put your phone away in your kitchen drawer after dinner or before your head off to bed, if it's safe to do so.
- Eat without a digital device on the table, in your pocket or by your side.

Self-compassion is the workout you need to build back this natural rest-and-recovery skill. When we do so, life really begins to wake up and we feel brighter and naturally more focused in the day.

You don't need permission to rest!

Discover the art of napping

I am a huge nap advocate! Naps are seriously underrated and often overlooked, yet they are an important building block in your sleep health.

Aside from pockets of recovery in our day away from busyess, the latest research shows that even a nine-minute nap has tremendous upsides for our focus, attention, brain and feelings of well-being without impacting our sleep appetite later on.[6] This is why naps in small, timed doses are such a useful recovery tool that can really help to boost alertness and help with cognitive fatigue (see page 184) as you switch from task to task in your everyday life.

Short naps are great for an afternoon boost. However, remember our sleep pressure builds from the moment we wake up (see page 66) and is a little bit like an appetite for sleep. If you sleep too long, you quell your appetite for sleep later at night. You may see conflicting advice about naps, but the best thing to remember is that short naps *at the right time* can be a great way to manage sleep stress and help you stay in a healthy rested state.

If you want to create a nap habit and give yourself a cognitive rest:

- Aim for a 10–20-minute nap ideally between 2 and 4pm. Just after lunch, our body temperature dips, which, coupled with the sensation of a full stomach, can make you feel quite naturally sleepy.
- Find a quiet place to sit or, even better, lie down. For those working from home, draw the curtains. (Increasingly, some offices and gyms are investing in nap pods for staff or have a prayer room or well-being space you can use.) Having a mini nap outside in a safe green space is a great alternative.
- Set an alarm to keep it short. More than 20–30 minutes can affect your next night's sleep.

IT'S ALL ABOUT HAVING A SHORT RECOVERY RESET NAP.

In a recent study published in the *European Journal of Sports Science*, researchers found that elite athletes were able to take short daytime naps and not suffer any adverse effects on their nocturnal sleep.[7] In what ways can your 'inner athlete' accept that rest protects and fuels your talent?

If you think you're rest-immune or unable to take a nap, the 'Rest Espresso Break' tool on page 139 is a great way to rest your eyes and activate a short recovery. It's also useful to know that any of the short breathing or relaxation mindset audios in this book are all very effective ways of calming down your stress system, giving you more choice in how you respond to your energy and working day, while also teaching you how to efficiently alternate between focused action and recovery.

SLEEP FOR WORKPLACE SUCCESS

In many studies, researchers found that those who had a short sleep at work scored better on tests of alertness and performance.[8]

Things have changed in the past five years and organisations are actually starting to think about sleep health policies. It's one of the most exciting areas of my work, helping to consult on and design sleep strategies for workers, all the way through to offering bespoke sleep one-to-ones. I know lots of leaders in businesses are now realising that afternoon performance is better after a short brain nap or core recovery period.

I'd like to introduce you to a couple of life's great athletes who might seem very different, but who have common goals:

Gus, an ultra-triathlete, came to me to learn how to micro sleep (or take a fast brain–body nap) in the miniscule gaps between races and thus enhance his performance along the way. He was keen to look after his sleep, recover better and learn how to settle down from huge surges of adrenaline. Ultimately, he needed to learn how to rest.

Every day, he trained and coached his mind and body into such high-energy states that initiating rest and sleep felt quite alien to him. Of course, he knew that adopting new rest techniques would create huge performance gains, relieve pressure and also help him look after his mental health.

This week's audio tools (page 214) changed everything for Gus. Every day, he practised and paid attention to relearning how, in just a few minutes, he could settle his nervous system and access calm, rest and active recovery. He taught himself how to take a short rest, anytime, anywhere. This was also useful for helping his approach to sleep at night because he practised the tools again as his head hit the pillow and if he happened to wake up earlier than planned. This simple repetition enabled him to make huge recovery gains.

Now meet Addy, the mother of a newborn baby, who wanted to learn how to reframe her rest in the face of stressed sleep. Having already navigated six weeks of extreme sleep deprivation while feeding her baby on demand, to me she was in her own ultra-athlete lane, feeling huge pressure, anxiety and the negative impact of poor sleep.

Understanding how daytime rest supports sleep was important in her recovery and the audio tools this week helped her to become confident about reclaiming her rest during the day. She hadn't understood that rest can be achieved in just a few moments.

ACTION: ACCESSING YOUR PERSONAL RECOVERY ZONE

When thinking about your personal recovery zone, it's highly beneficial to consider the natural and normal dips in your energy (your chronotype – see page 92) so that you don't corrupt your sleep at night. What does this look like for you? Can you focus this week on planning and timing that natural slow-down habit?

REST CAN BE ACHIEVED IN JUST A FEW MOMENTS.

HOW DAILY MOVEMENT SUPPORTS SLEEP

DAILY MOVEMENT = NATURAL NIGHT SLEEP 'MEDICINE'.

As we've seen, rest has been shown to be vital for reducing stress and achieving better sleep health. Exercise has also long been associated with better sleep and can promote better sleep quality in various ways:

- Exercising outdoors allows natural sunlight to fine-tune your circadian rhythm.
- Physical activity first thing in the morning and during the early afternoon can reset your sleep–wake cycle, allowing it to balance the production of cortisol and melatonin and, at night, trigger timely sleepiness to improve overall sleep quality.
- Daily movement prevents us from becoming too sedentary: an important consideration when, according to the Office for National Statistics, here in the UK the sedentary trend means that by 2030 we will be 35 per cent less active than we were in the 1960s.[9] Many people don't realise that daily movement and physical activity have significant benefits for our sleep health as well as our physical well-being.

There is no doubt that incorporating movement into your recovery each day is key to restoring balance and resetting your sleep health. It is also a helpful remedy for improving insomnia. Exercise is proven to be as effective as sleeping pills in relieving insomnia and research has shown that daily regular exercise of any kind can help chronic insomnia sufferers fall asleep up to 13 minutes faster and stay asleep for 18 minutes longer.[10] Exercise can also relieve the symptoms of anxiety and depression that are often the signature of confused and stressed sleep struggles.

EXERCISE IS A TWO-WAY STREET. SLEEP HELPS YOUR MOVEMENT AND MOVEMENT HELPS YOU SLEEP AT NIGHT.

The great news is that studies have shown that getting as little as ten minutes of aerobic activity per day is enough to significantly improve sleep quality.[11] In the sleep literature, movement is often defined as cycling, running and swimming. However, just remember that regular physical activity reduces the risk of insomnia and helps you get a restful night's sleep.

By the very nature of our mind–body connection, when we move we activate and flex our nervous system and breathing for the better.

Timing your exercise

When I am asked about the perfect time to exercise, I don't offer strict rules. It's completely personal to you, your current schedule and your sleep health goals. However, what is very clear is that both endurance and resistance training can enhance how quickly we fall asleep, how long we sleep for and the quality of our sleep. In my mind, all movement is beneficial for overall mind and body health and the reality is that most of us are not getting enough movement in our week.

Research shows that there are benefits to working out at different times of day, but it all depends on your goals, and of course, your chronotype.[12] If you choose to exercise in the early evening, you'll need to factor in a longer wind-down rather than falling into the 'can't sleep, won't sleep' insomnia thinking trap (see page 46). For example, if you've had a fast-paced day and load your evening with high-tempo exercise, you can't expect to easily wind down quickly to sleep. Think about the rhythm of your day – if you are doing higher tempo exercise such as high-intensity interval training (HIIT) or cardio, it will raise your blood pressure and core body temperature and be very alerting for your mind and body (which is, of course, not a bad thing if you are about to start a shift or have a complex work deadline due by 10pm!). Intense exercise also increases your adrenaline and cortisol levels, which makes you feel more alert, which is the last thing you want when you're trying to wind down for bed.

How movement helps your sleep

Cortisol regulation and sleep quality are connected.

Physical exercise modulates cortisol and sleep beneficially.

Light-to-moderate exercise is effective.

Exercise also increases the levels of endocannabinoids (neurotransmitters) in your blood, which can make you feel elated and full of energy. Late-evening cardio and strength work will almost certainly mean you need to hydrate close to bedtime, which could also disrupt your sleep.

Note to your inner athlete: if you have a scheduled training session or a match planned in the evening, you need to allow a longer wind-down or pre-sleep recovery afterwards to lead you into sleep. It's an excellent opportunity to do a Sleep Reset visualisation.

I want you to focus now on what your 'inner athlete' needs to succeed in life. Cast your mind back to the circadian science that we learned about in Week 2, where making the choice to expose yourself to bright morning light enables you to optimise your sleep health (see page 71). Think about the choices you can make that suit the rhythm of your day. Movement changes temperature and breathing, so, to make exercise as supportive to sleep as possible, you might choose to impose a two- to three-hour sleep protection window on any vigorous exercise that might disrupt your sleep wind down.

Mind–body exercises like some forms of yoga, Pilates and tai chi are relaxing to do in the late afternoon or evening and are great for relieving stress and setting the stage for you to get good deep sleep (see page 201–208).

Try to match your movement with when your daily energy peaks are. Think back to your chronotype, which we explored in Week 2 (page 92). By now, having made sleep, rest and recovery a priority, you should be finding yourself in harmony with your body clock. Working with your chronotype, the timing of your exercise or movement can really make an impact. If you want to become more of a 'morning' person, you can nudge your body clock by exercising and viewing daylight earlier. I'm a strong morning 'lark' and I aim to complete my exercise before midday when I can.

Morning exercise can help you reach your circadian daylight goals and shift your body clock and chronotype to help you become more of a morning person. An easy way to create this morning habit and become consistent is to start small. Can you manage five minutes before your shower or three minutes while your kettle boils, for example? Layering up from the smallest dose is the most effortless way to build this habit.

START STRONG, BUT SMALL AND EVERY DAY.

However, if you are an evening 'owl', synching your body clock to plan movement in the early evening instead of the morning will prevent any 'energy tension' (a term I use when coaching clients to help them recognise if they are working against instead of within their chronotype body clock typology – see page 92). While, of course, ideally we'd always try to work with rather than against our natural body clock to help us stay in balance, at times we have work demands or family or social commitments that mean this simply isn't possible. For example, sometimes we need to have better energy in the morning or, conversely, we'd like to feel less tired at night. Remember though, on the whole, the better we manage our energy, the less our stress thermometer increases and the better our ability to feel sleepy and wind down into good overnight sleep.

ACTION: COMMIT TO A REGULAR, TIMED MOVEMENT PRACTICE

If you are underslept and time-poor, but want to start exercising consistently (these are the people I help every day!), the first thing to remember is we never *find* time; we *spend* time.

Instead of adding five to ten minutes to your day pre-9am, what can you swap out in your daily life for consistent movement?

Below are some simple swaps you can try. Look for the answers in yourself: trust your wisdom to guide your self-awareness. What can *you* do differently?

- Kettle time: use the three minutes while the kettle is boiling to MOVE. Do some calf stretching, have your own silent disco or do some squats – whatever feels good for you. What will you choose to do in this time? Be definitive here for yourself – choose one strong thing.

- Steps over scrolling: can you choose a five-minute brisk walk over scrolling? Maybe try to add an extra one minute every day. Take an energising walk around the block – get the steps in where you can. You'll find that you can do this quite easily if you choose to step outside of familiar autopilot habits.

- Commuting power: can you get off the bus or train one stop early, walk to the station rather than taking your car or walk up and down the stairs rather than taking the lift? Extra movement can easily and effortlessly be integrated into your day.

- Take social walking breaks: these fuel feel-good connections, relieve stress and help calm your nervous system away from cortisol.

This week, aim to do exercise or movement at a consistent time of day for three or four days. This is an achievable and manageable starting point that allows you to reach your goals, moves you away from all-or-nothing thinking (see page 46) and offsets some of the health risks of poor sleep.[13]

Try to incorporate exercise habit cues into your day. My handheld weights are near my kettle and I have resistance bands in the fruit bowl in my kitchen and on the coffee table in my lounge. These tiny visual nudges help me make those small habit changes that are so beneficial for my sleep health and wider well-being.

'I don't enjoy getting up early to exercise before work. However, I enjoy exercise at the end of the working day as I find it's helpful in transitioning from "work" to "home". This is especially true on work from home days. Exercise isn't about flogging myself; it's about giving my body the opportunity to move, whether that is a walk, a run, a HIIT session or yoga. On days when I struggle for motivation, I ask myself: "Do I ever feel worse after exercise?" The answer is always a resounding no!'
Rebecca Levett, sports psychologist

FUTURE-PROOFING YOUR SLEEP WITH A WIND-DOWN ROUTINE

It's essential to remind yourself of the connections between mind and body through daily movement. In the sections below, we'll explore some easy ways you can build on your regular recovery methods with a good wind-down routine for a consistent mind–body reset.

Yoga
Yoga is largely defined in Western cultures as exercise – a flow of different yoga positions in a sequence of asanas (which focus on the physical body) and mudras (which focus on prana, or breath).

Personally, I think of yoga as a union of my mind, breath and body in motion.

Practising yoga not only has a physical effect; neuroscience shows that it leads to increased volume in brain regions responsible for our perception of pain tolerance and also helps the neuroplasticity of our mind–body connection.[14] When you consider that chronic pain and back pain are among the top five reasons for sleep disturbance, there's a compelling reason for making yoga a regular part of your routine.

Despite this, yoga is often overlooked as a serious sleep solution. Stretching is just one aspect of yoga; it also has profound body–brain benefits. The jury is out on which form of yoga is most potent for sleep from a science point of view – although hatha yoga, which focuses on body position, and nidra, which focuses on breathing and more restorative poses such as lying and seated postures, have great pre-sleep benefits. My advice is to explore different forms of yoga and find the style that you most enjoy and then build this into your Sleep Reset.

I know from personal experience how important yoga can be. My son, who has spina bifida, does a daily yoga practice to help his mobility and encourage his nervous system to strengthen weakened muscles. Yoga and mobility also play a starring role in the sleep retreats I host.

Yoga has been proven to alleviate symptoms of sleep apnoea (see page 222) and other sleep disorders and, time and time again, I see for myself in clinic how it becomes part of a weekly reset, a moving-forward strategy.[15] A particularly interesting study highlights that yoga is especially helpful for female sleep health, with the effects of yoga significantly improving sleep in women with sleep problems.[16]

Yoga engages certain regions of the brain responsible for processing our day-to-day environmental perception (the insular) and flexibility, while also helping areas of the brain shift more easily from sympathetic reaction (stress alertness) back down to our parasympathetic response (rest and digest) – see page 146. Understanding this brilliant constellation of mind and body benefits gives new meaning to your evening wind-down yoga or mobility routine. This is a perfect example of your nervous system, muscles and connective tissue working in harmony together with your thinking, focus and breathing.

Incorporating small, focused yoga movements into my own wind-down acts as an automatic cue to relax. I like to do yoga outside during the day whenever possible to get a circadian boost and, at night, I do yoga with my children before bed. When I don't do it, it also serves as an indication that I have become too busy.

Yoga movement and stretching both help ensure natural stress reduction, improved vagal tone and optimal functioning of body temperature, creating the balance we need to welcome sleep at night following our overstimulated, stressed days.

Pilates

I must admit to coming quite late to really appreciating Pilates for sleep. I hit a health hard stop with a cervical neck injury and had to rethink my movement practice for a whole year of my life. Having a regular Pilates dose in my week helped me gain back core strength and rehabilitate my back, but also helped me manage the pain and strengthen my spine. In my midlife, Pilates has been a really valuable recovery tool for my sleep well-being too and helps me promote balance and strength in my physical body.

Often our days are spent sitting at our desk or in our car, which leads to a poor, tense posture, especially for our head, neck and shoulders. Sitting all day tightens up our bodies, making it more difficult to physically release the day and sometimes creating the tension and discomfort we feel at night. Pilates moves, which include stretching and rolling, will help lengthen out every part of your body, opening up the joints, stretching the muscles and improving circulation, to name just a few of the physical benefits.

Pilates is also a practice that can easily become part of your pre-bedtime ritual, as well as a recovery practice during your day.

Studies have shown that Pilates decreases fatigue and has positive effects on sleep quality and emotional well-being.[17] One study also noted how being more connected to your body through Pilates is highly influential in being able to relax more.[18] Pilates is a promising new sleep wellness therapeutic intervention.

Spine-stretching movement sequences

A simple step towards building a bedtime recovery habit is to swap sleep-stealing scrolling for body-based scrolling – all in the comfort of your bedroom.

A slow movement stretching regimen is integral to good sleep health and can alleviate symptoms of sleep apnoea (which we'll explore on page 222). Mobility stretching activates the parasympathetic nervous system (see page 146 for more on this), which coaches your body to slow down, rest and digest, leading to good sleep and allowing your muscles to repair and regenerate.

The following short, simple, slow-paced bedtime stretching exercises may tempt you to build in this sleep health habit and ease your transition into sleep:

Restful bed legs

A restorative mobility pose that helps to reduce tension and provide release in your neck, back and shoulders while also promoting relaxation.

- Centre yourself and practise nose-breathing (see page 173) to regain your end-of-day focus.
- Sit with the right side of your body against a wall.
- Lie on your back and swivel to place your legs up against the wall. Your hips can be up against the wall too or a few inches away from the wall, as you prefer. You can also place a pillow under your hips for support and a bit of elevation if that helps.
- Rest your arms in any comfortable position, by your side or above your head.

- Release your neck in slow side-to-side movements – breathing in a steady state of awareness.
- Remain in this pose for five minutes and feel the reset effects.

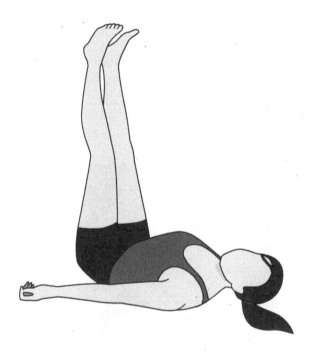

The bedtime roll-down and release-up
You can easily do this head into body roll-down in the comfort of your bedroom, making it a supportive recovery tool.

- To begin, stand with your back pressed against a wall.
- Let your head and arms slowly fold forwards, rolling yourself down one vertebrae at a time.
- When you have reached as far as is comfortable for you, hold for three seconds, then slowly roll back up. Repeat.

Bedtime bend and release

This is another beautifully simple position for releasing your neck and spine and setting yourself up for better sleep. This is also a brilliant way to 'unhunch' from the day.

- Sit down with your legs extended forward and reach out to touch your toes.
- Slowly inhale and exhale while in this position.
- Hold this pose for five cycles of breath and work towards maintaining this position for a restorative five minutes.
- Be creative, releasing back upwards and then mobilising slowly downwards again.

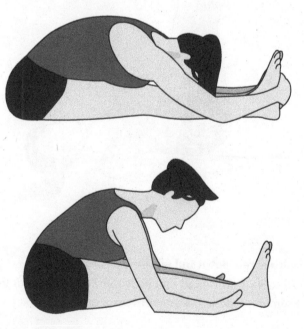

Tech neck shoulder release

This stretch is powerful in releasing screen-induced neck aches by conditioning the vagus nerve (see page 151).

- Use your hands to gently massage each side of your neck 15 times.

- Then rotate your neck, circling your head 15 times clockwise and then 15 times anti-clockwise.

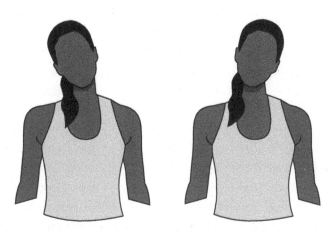

- Finally, circle your arms up and over to release the shoulders, 15 times forward and then 15 times backwards.

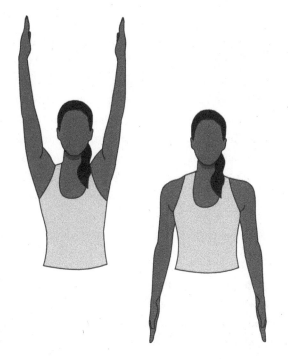

Shoulder rolls

These simple, rhythmic upper-body rolls can be done in bed with your legs crossed or stretched out.

* Think simple motion: simply roll your shoulders forward and then backwards.
* Then roll them up and down, hunching up tight and then releasing all the way down into a lengthened posture.

This routine will bring you closer to sleep health day and night. With these moves you will also be able to focus on breathing, which will calm the nervous system down, encouraging a more restful night's sleep and a more relaxed body to curl into bed. The same effect can be found with many mind–body practices such as tai chi (see below), with direct improvements in sleep well-being.

TAI CHI

Tai chi, as it is practised in the West today, is a moving form of yoga and meditation combined. When you perform tai chi, you complete a number of 'forms' - slow, graceful, fluid sequences of movements with smooth and even transitions between them.

One study in the scientific journal *Sleep* determined that the group who performed tai chi (compared to those who took classes on healthy lifestyles, including classes on sleep hygiene alone) had a significant improvement in the quality of their sleep, took less time to fall asleep, awakened less, slept longer and felt better rested.[19] This underlines my approach of how good sleep health connects both mind and body.

Don't forget to keep practising breathing exercises during the day so that you start to automatically breathe through your nose at night. Coupling this with the exercises above will have a positive impact on your sleep breathing.

FROM PILLOW TO PODIUM

The UK's most decorated Winter Paralympian team, Menna Fitzpatrick and Jennifer Kehoe, won four medals, including gold in the women's visually impaired slalom in the 2018 Winter Paralympics. Jen has a refreshingly relaxed approach to sleep under pressure:

'It's essential that I engage in the ritual of unwinding the tension in my body as part of my restful night's sleep. Daily physical and mental recovery helps me to maintain high performance levels throughout the long winter season.

'A typical bedtime routine would be to finish all my pre-bed admin like brushing my teeth, then make myself a warm milk with a hint of honey. Just before getting into bed I do five to ten minutes of gentle yoga, focusing on poses that relax me and holding them for longer than I would during a daytime practice. Usually this is enough to send me to sleep. If I've got a very busy brain, I love to listen to a relaxing audiobook.

'Lying in bed worrying about the fact I can't sleep has always seemed a bit pointless so I embrace familiar rest routines and allow myself a little more time to relax calmly and focus on my breathing into my positive mindset.'

This really illustrates that, even at the peak of performance, some sleep compassion and familiar routines for both mind and body and breathing can really help you sleep your biological best under pressure.

THE CHILLY DIP INTO GREATER SLEEP HEALTH

Back in 2018 I did my first lake triathlon and discovered the amazing sleep and well-being benefits of cold-water swimming. Since then, many well-regarded science journals have taken a closer look at the sleep and well-being benefits of deliberate cold-water exposure.[20]

So many studies show that exposure to cold water triggers and trains our stress response. This is called 'hormesis', a type of healthy stress that produces surprisingly positive health benefits and gives us the confidence and physical and mental ability to endure other stresses in the future.[21]

Cold- or cool-water swimming or ice immersion have tremendous nervous system, metabolic and sleep health benefits. It's scientifically proven that cold showers can do a whole lot of good for our mind and body, but also our sleep health if we get the timing right.[22] This is also true for ice tank immersion therapy at home or a good old cold-water bath dip. If you are one of the few people who hasn't yet heard of of the inspirational Wim Hof, do check him out (see Resources, page 267)!

Aside from the obvious exercise benefits, three sleep health benefits of daytime cool-water swimming include:

1. better quality sleep and stabilised cortisol rhythm
2. increased perceived happiness and positive self-regard
3. support for a resilient, healthy immune system

Cold-water immersion raises levels of hormesis, triggering cortisol and norepinephrine production. The changes in the brain also provide helpful chemical responses by activating the sympathetic nervous system and reducing inflammation.

Cortisol is involved in boosting alertness levels, and consequently if you time a swim for the morning or afternoon ONLY (as opposed to in the evening or late at night), you help the balance of that healthy wake–sleep cortisol arc and rhythm, remembering that cortisol levels in the body usually fall in preparation for sleep.

ACTION: **THE MORNING SHOWER BLAST**

This is a practical, science-based action and is something we can all make a choice to try to do.

Start small by trying a cooler shower blast in the morning or afternoon. It may take a couple of brave showers to become fully comfortable with this, but it is a sleep well-being and recovery tool that is free to do every day or if you feel tired after poor sleep. I promise it gets easier!

1. Enjoy one minute of your average warm shower temperature. It's a good idea to first wash your hair in this ambient temperature. Now for the fun part: relax and trust you're in full control.

2. Gradually turn the water temperature down to cool for 30 seconds as you turn away from the shower. You may want to begin as I did by heading in back and butt first, bracing yourself and your breath, or just placing your feet or legs underneath the water and then slowly moving your arms, torso and head under as you adjust to the chilly, energising blast!

Now you're ready for the brave recovery tool: I double dare you to health blast yourself with colder water for 30 seconds every day over the coming week. In time you will get used to this and crave it - trust me, it is like a hundred espressos and you will feel incredible afterwards.

Having a cold shower in the morning will make you more alert and anchor in a helpful temperature and circadian rhythm for your sleep well-being. However, despite all the great and deserving press about cold-water well-being therapy and immersion, a cooler shower at night will freshen and alert you, awakening your mind and body, making it trickier to fall asleep. Once our fight-or-flight response is stimulated, the stress hormone noradrenaline is released, which boosts our concentration and makes us feel alert. (Which, of course, can be of great use if you need to drive late at night or work a night shift.)

Remember that sleep is super sensitive to both body and environmental temperature, and we lose body temperature much more quickly in water than in air of the same temperature. It's therefore worth thinking about the water ritual you likely participate in every day – the night-time shower or bath. I know, for some, an evening shower can be a natural bookend to the working day and a useful wind-down into sleepy mode, but you may not have considered how the temperature can aid or delay your sleep and well-being.

COLD OR REALLY COOL WATER TOO CLOSE TO SLEEP TIME MAY DELAY FALLING ASLEEP.

Cool showers in the evening are alerting; warm baths are sleep-promoting and are scientifically proven as a sleep aid.[23] Warm-water immersion in a bath or a warm shower at night-time can benefit insomnia sufferers. A meta-analysis of 17 studies found that taking an evening shower or bath in warm water improves sleep quality.[24] Having a warm shower before bed paradoxically cools your core brain body temperature, which is super helpful for sleep.

For people suffering from insomnia, a warm shower or bath can also allow them to relax and prepare the mind and body for bed. Try adding essential oils for sleep to your bathing routine, which are proven to put you in a relaxed state and help you fall asleep.[25] Or get a diffuser and use sensory sleep well-being aromatherapy.

Zara has high energy and, when we first met, her routine as a fitness devotee included late-night HIIT to try to burn off energy, yet all it did was raise her core body temperature and prolong alertness. She was not making time for deliberate rest in her jam-packed evenings and sometimes needed to work late at home.

I suggested a more flexible reset and reshuffle of her evening routine that also recognised her desire for movement and exercise. This meant swapping her late HIIT and spin classes for a flowing, dynamic stretching practice before 7pm and a reduction in temperature and artificial light by taking a warm shower later in the evening by candlelight.

These gentle new night-time rituals, rooted in science-based biology, really gelled with Zara and allowed her to shake off the high-performance energy and adrenaline of her working day.

ACTION: LAYER IN A NEW WIND-DOWN HABIT

Can you embed a new evening ritual this week?

- Decide what sparked the most interest in movement for you: stretching, yoga, Pilates or even tai chi.

- Start small and focused: build a three-minute sequence into your bedtime routine.

- Can you use a warm night-time bath or shower to help you wind down at the end of the day?

You will be amazed at what a helpful body awareness reminder this is and, very quickly, with repetition, you'll be able to embed a five- to ten-minute non-negotiable way to close down the day and head into recovery mode.

This week, you have continued to boost your daytime recovery strategies and have learned the Sleep Reset rest skills that you can do anytime, anywhere to help you develop a new approach to sleep health. Leaving behind any judgement or pressure is key here to future-proof your sleep.

WEEK 5 SLEEP RESET TOOLKIT

In this last week of the Sleep Reset we end with a helpful reflection on what we have discovered about ourselves so far, guiding us to think about the ways we can keep making achievable, small changes that protect our sleep.

By now you've built up a huge sleep health toolkit. This week, I would like you to momentarily set aside this trusty toolkit and choose to just focus on the Week 5 recovery menu – three highly impactful audio tools designed to help consolidate your Sleep Reset journey in this final week.

YOUR WEEK 5 TOOLKIT RECOVERY MENU

1. Your Mindset Tool: Settle into the Recovery Flow Zone (5-minute guided audio download)

2. Your Breathing Tool: Deep Calm Ocean Breath (5-minute guided audio download)

3. Your Sleep Hypnosis: The Sleep Reset Mental Rehearsal (30-minute guided audio download)

Your Mindset Tool: Settle into the Recovery Flow Zone

Welcome to this next-level recovery mindset audio. The theme of this week is for you to see yourself as the inner athlete that you are. This tool allows you to shift gears with your breath at first and then build on your visualisation capacity. It also raises your confidence in finding helpful ways to train your mind–body muscle for recovery in the daytime.

Now is your chance to get serious about your daytime recovery gains. This audio tool guides you to practise moving towards your goals and is an effective reminder that recovery is an essential part of the process.

HOW THIS TOOL CAN WORK FOR YOU

This sleep mindset audio tool will:

- help to train your relaxation response

- protect your energy

- support you in practising nose breathing, which is better for sleep

---

This tool can wrap around (before or after) any mobility, movement or exercise that you accomplish this week. As this is an active relaxation, you can listen as you walk or move – but please don't do it while driving! It's an ideal sunset stroll reset tool too.

Top tip: this tool develops into a scan and progressive relaxation, so it's particularly effective in the evening after a heavy training session or a stressful day when you feel tense.

Your Breathing Tool: Deep Calm Ocean Breath

This is an easy-to-learn grounding breathing tool that will become your bedtime hero and is super useful if you can't sleep post-exercise or are busier than normal in the evening but want to feel sleepy.

Once learned, you can calm any breathing pattern into this sleep-help pace.

Top tip: get super creative and choose your favourite nature sound, chill-out or sleep wave playlist to listen to alongside this tool.

Your Sleep Hypnosis: The Sleep Reset Mental Rehearsal

This positive imagination sleep well-being guided tool is a wonderful way to celebrate a chapter of good sleep, soak in your complete

Sleep Reset journey and help keep you in that lovely sleep recovery zone.

Top tip: you can easily record this hypnosis in your own voice and update it along your personal journey. Use it as an everlasting Sleep Reset tool you can and will return to.

To make it easier for you to self-record, this sleep hypnotherapy transcript is hosted on www.mindtonicsleep.com.

YOUR WEEK 5 BONUS TOOLS

Celebrate

You have built such a strong foundation for your sleep, worked on your mindset and practised breathing. YOU have achieved this all for yourself. How can you celebrate this? What resonates for you?

Very often people take this renewed daytime energy and book in a day of radical self-care. Another easy way to celebrate your sleep health is to look back at the tips on optimising your sleep environment on page 28 and see what you can implement. Upgrading your sleep environment once you've done all the hard work is a nice way to future-proof your sleep.

YOUR REALISTIC SLEEP RESET 'PRESCRIPTION'

Congratulations on getting this far and repairing your relationship with sleep. This week, I suggest you focus on the Week 5 recovery menu to take your sleep health forward. You can build in the tools across the whole week or choose three or five days for a super-realistic approach. Alternatively, you can keep consistent with the tools and rhythm you have already set in motion.

Like so many people I have worked with, this week you may begin to feel the whole ripple effect of caring for your sleep health in this new, holistic way. It feels like a huge spring forward – your sleep has already been reset into great shape.

Tool	Monday	Tuesday	Wednesday	Thursday	Friday	Saturday (optional)	Sunday
Mindset							
Breathing							
Sleep Hypnosis							

COMMON SLEEP PROBLEMS

In this closing chapter we'll look more closely at common sleep problems, such as insomnia, sleep apnoea, Long Covid and hormonal changes, and the help that is on hand.

THE TOUGH NIGHTS OF INSOMNIA

The World Health Organization has pointed to a 'global epidemic of sleeplessness' with roughly two-thirds of adults sleeping fewer than eight hours a night. Various studies worldwide have shown the prevalence of insomnia in 10–30 per cent of the population, with some putting it as high as 50–60 per cent. In Europe, approximately one in ten adults suffers with chronic insomnia and the overall prevalence is increasing.[1] It is itself a sleep disorder, but is also one of the most prevalent sleep challenges that can creep up on us when our sleep feels stressed and we don't have the capacity to Sleep Reset.

Clinical insomnia (a sleep disorder in which you have trouble falling and/or staying asleep) can take us into our own personal 'pain cave' and amplify mental distress. I know this, intimately. I experienced many nights, weeks and even months of insomnia until I discovered the integrative mind–body approach that I've outlined in this book.

For far too long, many of us have been living with health symptoms caused by insomnia, which include, but are not limited to, a racing mind, difficulty falling asleep, waking up in the night or too early in the morning, daytime fatigue, irritability, brain fog, difficulty concentrating, depression and anxiety.

Here in the UK, it's widely reported that sometimes as many as a third of adults suffer from disturbed sleep each and every week. In my clinic, I focus on guiding those with chronic insomnia and I know this can be one of the loneliest afflictions, causing devastating effects on the body and mind.[2] In some cases, we can be caught up in an insomnia loop whereby not being able to sleep causes us to feel stressed, which in turn leads to us not being able to sleep. It can become the ultimate nightmare and, for some, this negative cycle continues for years without much respite.

The cycle of insomnia

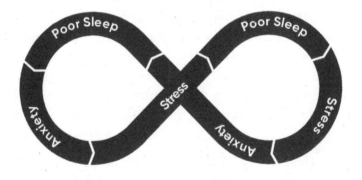

Insomnia is often diagnosed and quantified as enduring three nights of disrupted or barely any sleep in a week for a number of weeks. Chronic insomnia is defined as an inability to sleep at least three times a week for three months or longer. In my view, that is far too long to go without any support!

As we've seen, most people encounter sleep difficulties from time to time, often related to a new environment, stress or pain. Many of these bad sleep bouts get better without the need for treatment. However, your sleep issues may also be caused by a circadian rhythm disorder or you might suffer from chronic insomnia. Let's have a look at the difference between the two.

People suffering from circadian rhythm disorders are quite capable of falling asleep and staying asleep – it's just at completely the wrong time of day. This is because their body clocks are out of synch with their daily lives and environment, making them feel as if they are permanently jet-lagged.

There are a number of circadian rhythm disorders, including delayed sleep phase syndrome (when a person's sleep is delayed by two hours or more beyond what is considered a conventional bedtime), non-24-hour sleep–wake disorder (when an individual's biological clock fails to synchronise to a 24-hour day), jet lag and shift-work sleep disorder. Those with circadian rhythm disorders are commonly mislabelled as having insomnia; however, they are two separate issues.

If you believe you might be experiencing insomnia, firstly, it's important to establish if there is a medical reason causing it, so it's worth making a doctor's appointment as soon as possible while you work through the Sleep Reset. I always explain that, in its simplest form, insomnia is just a pattern. You were not born with it and, as with all the people I help, these patterns and behaviours can be worked through, supported and changed for better well-being.

LEARNING HOW TO ADVOCATE FOR YOUR SLEEP WELL-BEING IS EVERYTHING

Sadly, not enough people seek help with insomnia and I am on a mission to change that!

Remember, sleep problems and insomnia are very treatable and any increase in sleep quality impacts your emotional well-being and that whole brilliant circadian cascade we have explored in this book.

The first stop should always be to seek an urgent NHS face-to-face appointment if you can to talk about insomnia and your sleep health. One of the biggest mental barriers many people have when it comes to booking that first appointment with their

GP is that their sleep problem isn't 'bad' or 'serious enough' to warrant help and they can just struggle on.

That's just not true; it's always okay to ask for help and to seek out what sleep services are available to you. Your GP can also guide you to self-refer to any online sleep coaching or free resources. This can go hand in hand with the Sleep Reset, as the first steps you have taken in self-awareness and sleep compassion will really help.

INSOMNIA IS A PATTERN OF POOR SLEEP. YOU WERE NOT BORN WITH IT. IT CAN IMPROVE.

How the Sleep Reset can help

This book was not written to be an insomnia guide alone, but I have helped hundreds of insomniacs each year with this holistic Sleep Reset. If you've been diagnosed with insomnia and are waiting for an appointment with a sleep specialist, this whole book has been designed as a supportive helping hand to guide you through. You can make the choice to start in Week 1 and run through the five-week method chronologically, or you can use the book in an intense way and treat each week as a single day – so a five-day Reset – to really help support yourself.

Even if there is a medical cause for your insomnia, behavioural conditioning can still be your best defence against it and is a proven helping hand back to better sleep. For many of my patients, this approach can provide a route out of helplessness and a practical way of supporting their sleep.

Sleep really is in the mind and body. Everything you do, think and feel is linked, and understanding this relationship holds the key to sleep-promoting thoughts and beliefs that, in turn, will help to positively shape your recovery from insomnia. No matter what is disturbing your sleep, it's important to engage in behaviour that helpfully promotes good sleep. Look back to Week 2 and the solid foundation of consistency for your body clocks and the good practice of morning light and evening dark – this is what good behaviour that supports high-quality sleep looks like.

Daily movement is also a helpful remedy for improving insomnia (see Week 5). Exercise is proven to be as effective as hypnotic drugs in relieving insomnia, bestowing quality sleep rather than the sedated 'junk' sleep that many hypnotics can give you.[3]

SLEEP RESTRICTION

In some cases, clinically guided sleep restriction when working with a sleep therapist or practitioner one to one can be a useful deeper sleep tool for insomnia. Please advocate for yourself and speak to your GP if you think this might be something you'd like to explore.

SLEEP APNOEA

Obstructive sleep apnoea (OSA), the most common type of sleep apnoea, typically occurs when the muscles that support the throat, including your tongue and soft palate, relax too much to allow normal breathing. These muscles support structures including the back of the roof of your mouth (soft palate), the triangular piece of tissue hanging from the soft palate (uvula), the tonsils and the tongue.

When the muscles relax, your airway narrows or closes as you breathe in, hampering your breathing for ten seconds or longer. This can lower the level of oxygen in your blood and cause a build-up of carbon dioxide.

Your brain senses this impaired breathing and briefly rouses you from sleep so that you can reopen your airway. You can awaken with shortness of breath that corrects itself quickly, within one or two deep breaths. You might make a snorting, choking or gasping sound. This awakening is usually so brief that you don't remember it.

This pattern can repeat itself 5–30 times or more each hour, all night long. These disruptions lead to fragmented sleep, impairing your ability to reach the deep, restful phases of sleep, and you'll probably feel sleepy during your waking hours. Disturbed sleep makes you feel permanently groggy and tired, impacting your daily life and activities, everyday chores, work and even your ability to drive. With this in mind, it's important to understand the condition and what you can do to ease it.

There's also central sleep apnoea, where the brain fails to send the correct signal to your body to inhale, causing you to miss a breath or multiple breaths in succession. And finally, there's mixed sleep apnoea, a combination of both the above.

Anyone can develop OSA. However, certain factors put you at increased risk, including:

- Gender: in general, men are twice or three times as likely as premenopausal women to have OSA. The frequency of OSA increases in women after menopause.
- A family history of sleep apnoea.
- Asthma: research has found an association between asthma and the risk of OSA.
- Narrowed airway: you might inherit naturally narrow airways, or your tonsils or adenoids might become enlarged and block your airway.
- High blood pressure (hypertension): OSA is relatively common in people with hypertension.
- Chronic nasal congestion: OSA occurs twice as often in those who have consistent nasal congestion at night, regardless of the cause. This may be due to narrowed airways.
- Smoking: people who smoke are more likely to have OSA.
- Very high body mass index (BMI): not all people with OSA are overweight, but a wide neck with fat deposits around the upper airway can obstruct breathing.

- Older age: the risk increases as you age but appears to level off after your 60s and 70s.
- Diabetes: OSA might be more common in people with diabetes.

OSA tended to be more common in midlifers and skewed towards males, but new research on OSA illustrates that this isn't exactly the case.[4] It's now thought that perhaps OSA is hugely underdiagnosed, with increased diagnoses occurring in young children, teens and also in females.[5] A recent study published in the *Journal of Clinical Sleep Medicine* revealed that women often don't seek the help they need (see box below for more on female sleep apnoea).[6]

The classic primary hallmarks of OSA are snoring and excessive daytime sleepiness, but waking up with a dry mouth and feeling excessively thirsty are also often reliable clues. It's useful to remember that some symptoms happen when you're asleep, and others when you're awake. Naturally there will always be a broad range of symptoms and not everyone with OSA will experience all of them. Conversely, just because you are experiencing a few symptoms doesn't necessarily mean you have OSA.

FEMALE SLEEP APNOEA

Across sleep research it appears that, once again, female sleep health hasn't been given the spotlight it deserves, especially when it comes to sleep breathing disorders. While men are more likely to experience the 'classic' symptoms of OSA mentioned above, women who are eventually diagnosed with OSA often display different non-specific symptoms, such as headaches, sleep struggles and anxiety.

The few population studies that have included women show that undiagnosed OSA is far more prevalent in women than men. One study found that OSA was undiagnosed in more than 90 per cent of women with moderate-to-severe OSA.[7] I want to highlight this so that you can advocate for yourself if you have started snoring or have any of the other symptoms associated with OSA and can speak to your GP about an early referral to your local sleep study.

OFTEN SNORING IS YOUR BODY'S 'BEIGE FLAG' TO SEEK HELP, SO IT'S ESSENTIAL YOU USE THE SLEEP RESET ALONGSIDE SOME CLINICAL SLEEP SUPPORT.

PCOS is a risk factor too. I have PCOS, so I was interested to learn that women with this endocrine disorder may be at higher risk due to an excess of male hormones, which are linked to snoring and sleep apnoea, and are already at increased risk of insomnia.[8] Aside from PCOS, there are other medical conditions that are associated with OSA, such as asthma, metabolic syndromes, hypothyroidism and obesity.

It's a common myth that only people with a high BMI are at risk. In fact, sleep disorders also tend to overlap, and patients with OSA may suffer from comorbid insomnia, circadian (internal body clock) disorders, sleep movement disorders (like RLS) and/ or conditions of hypersomnia (such as narcolepsy).

If you're one of the 4 million people in the UK suffering from sleep apnoea, actually obtaining that all-important shut-eye is anything but restful.[9] You might suffer from loud or laboured breathing while sleeping or feel as though your breathing isn't regulated, causing unpleasant gasping sensations that interrupt rest and repair for your body and mind.

Too many people don't make the connection between loud, disruptive snoring, long pauses in breathing, repeated night-time awakenings, unrefreshing sleep, insomnia, trouble thinking or excessive daytime sleepiness and mild OSA, and instead just focus on the hours of sleep alone and muddle along. (Snoring can also be caused by excessive weight around the middle, lack of exercise and dehydration, and it is also worsened by caffeine and alcohol.) If any of this relates to you or a loved one, seek sleep well-being help and advocate for your sleep health as soon as possible.

If you suspect you have OSA or a sleep disorder, the most important advice I can give you is to seek professional or medical help, especially if your symptoms appear to be getting worse. Push your GP to take your sleep health seriously and get them to assess your symptoms and, if needed, refer you to a sleep clinic or sleep specialist. To really improve a patient's sleep and daytime functioning, a detailed sleep-related history and an individualised behavioural sleep medicine approach is needed. A CPAP machine (a device that gently pumps air into a mask you wear over your mouth or nose while you sleep at night) could also be a solution. (You'll be given this for free on the NHS if you need it in the UK.) See also Resources, page 265.

Taking empowered control of your sleep health starts right here. Below are some simple ways to manage sleep apnoea:

Reset your sleep position
Sleeping on your side helps by using gravity to open the airway. It's worth noting that when it comes to sleeping positions, sleeping on your back is easily the most unhelpful for sleep breathing disorders as gravity works against you, making breathing dysregulated.

Try sleep aids
A low-tech yet highly effective sleep aid is the mandibular advancement device, which looks a bit like a gum shield or mouth guard, and is something your GP or dentist can refer you to a specialist for. It's worn while you're sleeping to help keep your airway open and ensures breathing becomes easier.

For an easily accessible, off-the-shelf sleep aid, you might want to try mouth breathing tape – which involves fixing porous tape over both the upper and lower lips so that you cannot easily open your mouth, thereby prompting nose breathing while sleeping – which also encourages and drives up sleep quality. I started using mouth tape and have subsequently learned to unconsciously breathe in a far better, more functional way for health and well-being.

However, when asked what I am most excited about in the sleep aid world, without hesitation, it's the AcuPebble SA100 (see Resources, page 271). The first medical device to obtain the CE mark for automated diagnosis of OSA, it was developed at Imperial College London by a stellar all-female team led by Professor Esther Rodriguez-Villegas. It's not overstating things to say that this is a breakthrough in at-home monitoring sleep medicine that I'm proud to champion, and one that will help primary care support sleep more easily.

This device enables you to take accurate readings of your sleep breathing, respiratory patterns and heart rate, enabling you to detect sleep apnoea without a lab or intrusive equipment over a number of nights. I used it myself as I was concerned that I might have developed OSA after surgery. I carried out night readings over two weeks, which happily confirmed that I don't snore and don't currently have a sleep breathing disorder.

Practise deep breathing

Mind–body integrative practices, such as transformational yogic breathing, can benefit those who suffer from sleep apnoea by addressing oxygen levels within the body. Deep, meditative breathing helps improve the body's ability to circulate and absorb oxygen, creating feelings of calmness before bedtime, which is ideal if your disorder is causing anxiety before you even place your head on the pillow!

A review of 14 studies on the effects of breath retraining (a clinical term for breath conditioning exercises to help you breathe better during sleep) and the regular practice of breath control activities, including singing and playing wind instruments, concludes that they can potentially help sleep apnoea.[10]

ACTION: TONING YOUR MUSCLES FOR BETTER SLEEP BREATHING

Workouts shouldn't be restricted to exercising the usual muscles in your body. Giving smaller muscles, specifically those in your mouth, throat, soft palate and tongue, a daily workout to strengthen and tone them can work wonders. Strengthening the muscles we use to breathe may help them maintain more tension during sleep, in turn keeping your airways open and reducing sleep apnoea.

Tongue stretch

- Choose to start toning the muscles in your tongue by stretching your tongue out as far as you can.

- Try touching your chin with your tongue while you look up.

- Hold for ten seconds and repeat five times.

Tongue slide

- Choose to put your tongue on the roof of your mouth right behind your front teeth.

- Slowly slide your tongue back along the roof of your mouth.

- Repeat this exercise five times.

- If doing this exercise at night, repeat 20 times.

Tongue push-up

- Choose to push your entire tongue up against the roof of your mouth.

- Rest and hold for ten seconds and repeat this exercise five times.

Tongue push-down

- Choose to begin with the tip of your tongue touching the front of your lower teeth, push your entire tongue flat against the bottom of your mouth and allow it to rest.

- Hold it for ten seconds and repeat five times.

End-of-day release and yell

- Open your mouth wide and stick your tongue out as far as possible in a downward position like a lion roaring (it feels weird but is highly effective)!

- The uvula – the small fleshy piece at the back of your throat – needs to lift upwards as you stick your tongue out.

- You can choose to use a mirror to ensure that you're raising the uvula correctly. (Eventually, you will be able to sense the uvula lifting naturally.)

- Hold the elevated uvula for five seconds and repeat ten times.

How the Sleep Reset can help

All the sleep breathing tools are a brilliant support for you, but make sure you've covered the strong foundations of the Sleep Reset and worked through the weeks in order.

NEURODIVERGENT STRUGGLES

This is a subject very close to my heart. We are a neurodiverse family and I also work to champion and support sleep health for neurodivergent communities.

Sleep problems are a characteristic feature of children with autism spectrum disorder (ASD) with 40–80 per cent experiencing sleep difficulties.[11] Sleep problems have been found to have a pervasive impact on a child's socio-emotional functioning, as well as on parents' psychological functioning.[12]

While sleep troubles at times are universal, research shows that some neurodiverse people tend to struggle more frequently.[13] We typically see complex bedtime routines and difficulty winding down, making it easier to fall into distraction habits that fuel really late bedtimes, night waking and early-morning waking, which especially impact upon the daytime quality of their life and that of their families.

Approximately 50–80 per cent of children with ASD will display sleep problems compared to 9–50 per cent of children with typical development.[14] Sleep disturbance in children with ASD remains poorly understood but is thought to be a mix of biological, psychological, social/environmental and family factors.

A sleep disturbance is considered to be present when one or more of the following occur five or more nights per week:

- bedtime resistance problems
- delayed sleep onset
- sleep association problems
- night-time awakenings
- frequent early-morning awakening

This lack of sleep can impact in the following ways:

- increased sensitivity to stress/sensory overload
- increased stress, which can lead to meltdowns, thereby fuelling tension, anger and aggression
- emotional instability
- hyperactivity, changes to energy
- increased behavioural problems
- irritability and lethargy, low mood
- poor learning and cognitive performance in education settings and at home
- difficulty sticking to healthy coping strategies for parent and carer

How the Sleep Reset can help

The Sleep Reset and its realistic support tools have been incredible in my work to help my own neurodiverse teens and the many families and communities I support. Self-compassion is key here to dealing with the inevitable daily sleep–wake challenge and potential tensions.

Sleep is very often a sensory – nervous system – experience and we can harness this to our advantage if we switch attention to the sensory experience of our sleep time and sleep room. My top tip would be to really consider sound. Do you prefer sound-masking or do you like white or pink noise – ASMR – as a useful sleep distraction?

Also have a think about light and look back at Week 2 for some effective strategies to utilise natural daylight and evening light to optimise your sleep health. Some neurodiverse people like the comfort of a small red cosy light or indeed a super-dark cave-like room free from all clocks and time distractions. Consider your own sensory profile here.

I worked with Jay, who had recently been diagnosed in his twenties as having ASD and ADHD. Jay described his evening mind as being pretty rowdy and found it almost impossible to have a daytime sleep or nap. We therefore tailored his Sleep Reset to focus on mobility/stretching while he supported training his busy mind with sleep hypnotherapy. He accepted that, for him, a one-hour wind down (see page 81) instead of his rushed 15-minute pre-bed ritual was non-negotiable. We switched from him scrolling on his phone to having nature TV in his Sleep Reset (remember, there is no judgement here on screen time, just realistic choices you can make for your own sleep health). This helped him ease what he calls his 'fast rocket' brain more gently into bed instead of fuelling frustration.

WEIGHTED BLANKETS

Weighted blankets are an important and helpful new sleep intervention (see Resources, page 272). Research has shown that a weighted blanket could help you achieve satisfactory sleep, including improved sleep-onset latency, sleep continuity and sleep routines, and achieve overall well-being, including improved relaxation and reduced anxiety.[15] They are used frequently by children and adults with ADHD and/or ASD. Experiencing the relaxation of deep pressure sensory stimulation (touch) may create calming effects as a result of calming the central nervous system.

LONG COVID

Thankfully, my field of health care is beginning to understand more about the devastating impact Long Covid can have on sleep health. During any illness it's common to sleep more as your body fights an acute or chronic infection. Infection often affects sleep patterns and you may find yourself experiencing periods of longer and deeper than usual sleep when you fall ill. Other key hallmarks include extreme fatigue and insomnia. There are many reasons why your sleep might have changed after you had Covid-19 or while experiencing Long Covid. Medicine used to treat infections can very often affect your sleep and the change in your behaviours through being poorly very often takes you away from the circadian cues of light, movement and timing of food.

Rebecca came to me after many months of feeling defeated by different approaches to her Long Covid. She felt she had very little energy to keep trying new things after being bounced around various consultants and clinics. Her mental wellbeing was taking a huge downturn as she grappled with wanting to protect her precious energy but also feeling frustrated at being stuck indoors. She intuitively wanted to strip things back and look for a more holistic approach to recovery – starting with her sleep. She wanted to enjoy her bed and not feel like she was always in this twilight zone.

We worked through the Sleep Reset together across the five weeks and she particularly found the breathing and sleep hypnosis tools to be really potent for her as they required only gentle, low-energy effort. These recovery tools were something she could do that helped promote a sense of well-being and, layered together, worked to support her healing journey.

How the Sleep Reset can help

Your circadian sleep system needs natural daylight and then darkness to help you feel sleepy – being ill in bed at home or in hospital may mean that you have not got any natural daylight and have had changes to your daily patterns of movement and eating habits. All of these are sleep well-being cues to your body clock.

I asked one particular client with Long Covid: 'Where do you spend most of your time and what is the quality of light in that environment?' She knew the answer: it was immediately obvious that the safety and comfort of her sofa, her habitual sleeping place, was missing all the circadian-boosting natural light we learned so much about in Week 2. A little self-compassion also stopped her tendency to stress about her day in its tracks.

This is not about fixing Long Covid, but the 'Calming Box Energy Reset' (page 54) and the 'Deep Calm Ocean Breath' (page 214) tools can help you regain some elements of control and offer gentle support. When working with clients suffering from Long

Covid, I explain that self-compassion is very often a potent and undervalued quality. The sleep breathing tools can be practised at any time and help to break through the cycle of health anxiety and stress exhaustion.

The key elements of the Sleep Reset – self-awareness and the science-based audio mind and body tools – are a massive support to anyone facing sleep turbulence, natural anxiety and the sleep challenges caused by chronic fatigue or Long Covid.

I'm heartened at the attention being paid to continuing research around Long Covid as we begin to understand more about the impact this debilitating condition can cause.[16]

SLEEP HEALTH AND YOUR IMMUNITY

We have known of the links between poor sleep and our immune system for a while, but Covid-19 brought global attention to the importance of our immune function.

Sleep can help boost the immune system and can even prevent you from getting sick.[17] Your immune system will automatically do its very best for you if you give it an opportunity to be supported by sleep. You need to protect it by keeping to a regular sleep-wake circadian rhythm as we looked at in Week 2.

Our immune system has three layers of protection: the skin, the innate (the immune system you were born with) and adaptive systems. The adaptive part of the immune system creates a memory of prior infection, thereby producing antibodies as a protective measure if it returns. Cytokines (small proteins crucial in the growth of immune cells) are part of the innate system and send little SOS signals to recruit both killer cells and white blood cells.

We can get infections from the external world via our eyes, nostrils, mouth and ears, which can spike our immune system, but did you know that mindful breathing (where you guide your breathing into a slow, steady rhythm as you have been doing with the tools) has been shown to enhance the immune system, combat stress, fight illness and improve our sleep health?[18]

Our mindset and thinking can also have a direct influence on healing and inflammation. As we have already explored, we have multiple mindsets, and these can have a positive effect on our fully connected mind and body and our breathing.

Our brilliant circadian body clocks regulate how our immune system functions; this is particularly important to know for those in the frontline and healthcare settings whose sleep may be disrupted due to shift work or lack of exposure to natural daylight.

You are four times more likely to catch a winter bug after just one week of short sleep (around six hours of sleep or less each night) and are much more susceptible to common coughs and colds.[19]

You can look at this as strong motivation to stay with the supportive tools of the Sleep Reset. We can all enhance our immune system. Looking after your sleep helps look after your immunity, no matter what your gender or age.

THE NIGHT SHIFT NEED-TO-KNOW

Extreme circadian instability experienced by shift workers such as medics, nurses, doctors and factory workers can cause a variety of chronic health problems quite apart from poor sleep. It makes establishing regular daily patterns more challenging and can swiftly erode our emotional well-being and resilience.

As a shift worker you really are a sleep hero in my eyes. You are at the sticky end of sleep, but that is all the more reason to gift yourself the very best Sleep Reset that you can. Getting through the first night of your night shift is usually easier than the second or third night as fatigue begins to set in, particularly if you are having difficulty sleeping.

All the tools in this book will help you in some way (the only one that you can't harness is, of course, a consistent wake-up time). I've also included some tips specific to shift work below:

Schedule a circadian break

Look back at Week 2 where we discussed the circadian rhythm and body temperature. The time when the core body temperature is at its lowest is between 3am and 6am. Night-shift workers may naturally experience this hard-wired circadian cooldown at this time, with feelings of being tired, cold, shaky, nauseous, sleepy and drowsy. This is a normal reaction as the body is programmed to be less active at this time. It can be difficult to stay awake, especially if work demands are low.

If this is you, if possible, try to schedule a break during this time and plan a healthy coping response for it. Eat and drink something warm (avoid caffeine) and try to keep busy if a break isn't possible.

Train your nap rhythm

Try as much as you can to schedule naps and stick to the same times and length of time each day. Consistency is key here; our bodies love and thrive on rhythm so, by sticking to a regular nap time as much as possible, you will improve your sleep. Try a short, protected, scheduled nap of less than 30 minutes, especially before and during work shifts (if possible).

The Royal College of Physicians' shift-working guidance for junior doctors allows for power naps and calls it 'an indispensable part of working safely overnight'.[20] This is how essential napping can be for the safety of everyone on the ward, especially for protecting your mental well-being and patient care.

Avoid stimulants and sedatives

Shift workers often rely on caffeine crutches and alerting stimulants such as strong coffee and high-energy drinks to keep them awake, and alcohol or sleeping pills to help them sleep. The effects of both stimulants and sedatives are only short term and will lead to stressful sleep health. Try to avoid depending on either as a long-term strategy for dealing with shift work. Meditation, audio/sound stimulation or music therapy are way better than stimulants or sedatives.

Diarise your sleep

The number one thing I see when working alongside shift workers is that sleep is not blocked out enough in their diaries. It sounds obvious, but in this busy world, there is always something teasing at your scrolling eyes that sneakily snatches the odd 30 minutes of sleep here and there across your shift. Plan in your sleep time and schedule small doses of daily exercise – use them like your well-being anchors.

Block your Sleep Reset intention in your diary, stick it on the fridge or record a voice note of your self-compassion statement on page 37.

Plan your meals

Meal planning, or at least healthy snack and hydration planning, goes a long way to helping you with sleep success. Ideal snacks to encourage sleep are dairy- and carbohydrate-rich foods containing tryptophan (see page 109), such as bananas, nuts and seeds, milk, eggs, honey, low-fat cheese and yoghurt. Also, make sure you consume enough magnesium in your diet (found in meat and dark leafy green veg) as this essential mineral helps us sleep (see page 117).

Develop a bedtime ritual

Routine is everything. Look back at page 201 and develop a bed-time wind-down ritual that you follow before you go to sleep – relax with a book, listen to music or take a bath. Really zoom in on those mind-coaching cues and send familiar signals that this is the time to be ready for sleep and recovery.

Double down on the advice on page 28 on optimising your

sleep environment. It is far easier physiologically to fall asleep in a cool room over a warm/hot room. Keep your bedroom as cool as possible – around 16–18°C.

It may be harder in the day to keep the home and bedroom quiet, so do not be afraid to use sound-softening earplugs that help muffle, but not block out, sound. Also try an eye mask if necessary.

Don't abandon your social life

It's essential that you don't struggle alone. It may sound simple, but we often overlook our 'village of support' when we're tired. Chat to co-workers about sleep – sharing your Reset journey and meaningful goals will really help. Recruit support everywhere you can, especially during downtime. It will help you do the basics really well.

Your social and emotional well-being is hugely important. Try to continue having as much of a social and family life as possible. Make family and friends aware of your shift schedule so that they can include you when planning social activities.

Advocate for your employee rights

In the UK, you should have a minimum of 20 minutes' break away from the work environment if the shift is longer than six hours.[21] If you are unable to take your break away from the work environment during a night shift, then you should discuss this with your manager.

STRATEGIES TO ADOPT DURING THE SHIFT

- Eat regularly: try to eat your main meal before going on shift and have lunch halfway through the shift and another light meal when you get home. Eating small amounts often throughout the night will keep your energy levels up. Find out what works for you, but avoid a heavy meal before going to sleep.

- Mobilise your shift with micromovements: keep moving during the shift; if you have downtime, walk about and stretch.

- Wind down into a shift caffeine holiday: keep hydrated, but don't drink too much caffeine (see pages 125–131 for more on this). Try a pattern of night shifts with HALF the caffeine you had before, tapering down to none during the 3–6am window as best you can. This will really help your sleep because of the long caffeine tail (see page 125).

- Get home safely at the end of a night shift: if you are driving to and from work, be super aware of the risks of fatigue driving. Avoid driving for long periods or a long distance after a period of night shifts or long working hours.

GETTING BACK INTO A NON-NIGHT-SHIFT PATTERN

- Try your best to avoid getting a big chunk of sleep during the day and just have one sleep cycle (90 minutes). Take a short nap instead, ideally before midday – timing matters.

- When you wake up, see if you can eat, get outside and then consider a short burst of exercise (this alerts you and helps you wake up). Try to mimic a typical day's pattern as much as possible.

- Give yourself some self-compassion and know that it takes TIME! It's completely normal to take two to three days to readjust when you come off nights as you naturally allow your circadian system and body clocks to re-establish your typical awake in the day and sleeping at night pattern.

Nursing department head Nicky, a night-shift worker, describes her sleep issues below in her own words:

'Many of us confess to necking Night Nurse on a Friday after work purely as sedation to get to sleep, but Saturday morning would entail a hellish hangover which dominated my precious few days off. Far from feeling rested, a vicious cycle took hold which ruined any sense of recovery for me. I did what many of us do and pushed on, but the stress was deep inside and very loud as my head hit the pillow each night.

'The Sleep Reset has been a revelation. I have finally achieved sustained sleep throughout the night for the majority of the week and have also managed to get back to sleep really easily when I do wake.

'The breathwork has been vital in helping me focus back into rest when I wake in the night and has been just as valuable during the day, grounding me when I need to step back and literally take a breath. I've tried to settle into a daily routine where I stop and do some deep breathing periodically, which helps me focus and retain concentration for longer periods, energising my mind.

'I listen to the audios each evening after I finish work to unwind and settle. These behavioural therapies have played an integral part in improving my sleep and uplifting my sense of mental well-being. Far from being an exercise in self-indulgence, this has become a form of survival and a way of life, helping me act in a calmer, more measured way and making for a better work–life balance.'

UTILISING YOUR BODY TEMPERATURE FOR SHIFT WORK OR JET LAG

The concept of temperature minimum is really helpful when you experience shift work or jet lag. We tend to be sleepy when our body temperature is falling and we feel more alert as it is rising.

Sleeping and waking are directly tied to our temperature, which has a daily high (about 8-12 hours after waking) and a daily minimum (about 1.5-2 hours before your average wake-up time).

For me, this looks like:

My unique wake-up time: 6am

My temperature minimum: 4.30am

Knowing this 4.30am temperature minimum is my anchor point and helps me advance my clock if I need to go to bed later or earlier and can help me plan for shift work or travel.

Research has shown that if we view bright light in the four to six hours *after* our temperature minimum, we will push our circadian clock to regulate and 'phase advance', which wakes us up a little earlier and supports us to feel healthily alert, awake and energised.[22] Viewing bright light four to six hours *before* our temperature minimum will push our circadian clock to wake us up later the next day.

JET LAG TROUBLESHOOTING

Jet lag is a temporary sleep disorder resulting from the effects of travelling across different time zones. If your destination is only a time zone or two away, you may need to make only minor adjustments. However, when we journey long distances, perhaps flying across several time zones, few of us can avoid the effects of jet lag – feeling out of sync and fatigued.

Jet lag is the confusion between your internal body clock and the actual time, and the effects get much worse when you're travelling east as you're losing time. Many frequent flyers travelling west find this an easier adjustment because the day is lengthened rather than squeezed. It's easier to stay up later than it is to suddenly try to go to bed really early.

The further you travel and the greater the time difference, the more acute the impact is likely to be, especially if you are crossing more than three times zones or travelling east across the globe.

The human body clock will gradually readjust to a new time zone and symptoms usually improve within a few days, though a rule of thumb is that it takes one day per time zone going west to adjust and 1.5 days per time zone if travelling east.

One of the most common travel-related sleep stress experiences is known as the 'first night effect' – feeling restless or experiencing travel sleep insomnia. So many of us experience significant trouble when sleeping in a new and unfamiliar environment. It's useful to remember there's a biological reason why some of us won't experience a deep, quality rest or be able to sleep as soundly as hoped on the first night. Scientists have discovered that we sleep 'on alert' when we first arrive in a new environment.[23] Part of our brain stays more alert to 'keep watch' in case of danger, so it's perfectly natural to experience some first night sleep turbulence, but you can take back control of your sleep when you wake in the morning and help to encourage a better night's sleep the next day.

It's useful to take a 360-degree approach to jet lag, taking into consideration both mind and body. It's amazing how quickly shifting your perspective and following helpful lifestyle factors including eating nutritious food, increasing movement and ensuring mental rest and rejuvenation can help your body adjust to jet lag.

Below are my top tips to minimise and recover from jet lag:

Plan your meals

It's a good idea to time when you eat to suit your adjusting body clock so you feel your best for any holiday activities you have planned. Food can be a powerful way to stay energised, harness your energy effectively to feel at your peak when it's needed most and acclimatise to jet lag, even if you feel too tired or wired to eat.

Remember that your circadian rhythm is influenced by the timing of food, so use food as a cue to your body that it is time to stay awake if suffering from jet lag.

Light relief

Harness the magic of natural daylight and get out into the early-morning sun. Natural daylight is your best source of energy and most potent ally to cope with jet lag.

Although it's so important to protect your eyes from UV damage in the sunshine, it can be helpful to ensure there are occasions (such as when you first arrive) when you don't block out the sun with heavy dark glasses as it may hinder your recovery from impending jet lag. A little exposure to natural daylight can be helpful to let your body naturally adjust too.

Reduce the booze

For some, it's normal to feel celebratory when on a plane for leisure or even work, having a glass or two to toast your trip, or to dramatically increase your intake of caffeine for those early flights, but this will dehydrate you fast and worsen the symptoms of jet lag as your body recovers best when it isn't depleted of fluids.

Try to keep alcohol, coffee and energy drinks to a minimum and instead opt for a far better choice – water for ultimate hydration.

Hack the clock

Another effective travel well-being hack is to change your watch, phone or laptop to match the time of your chosen destination when you first get on board as this will mentally prepare you for the new time zone.

Get on the move

Exercise upon landing is essential to help you cope better with the symptoms of jet lag. Moving lightly with a gentle jog or even just a brisk walk outside in natural daylight will help to boost your sense of well-being and combat feelings of tiredness and poor cognition.

Create a home away from home

Taking a sense of the familiar away with you can help set your bedtime routine. Something as small as a favourite scent or a treasured photo can create a sense of safety and peace of mind, leading to a better sleep environment while away from home.

One must-have for me (if I have enough room) is to take my favourite pillow, so I can ensure the same level of support and comfort for my head and neck that I'm used to at home.

INFRARED SAUNA

This little-known sleep health therapy may be worth exploring or at least learning about for your personal sleep health.

Infrared sauna is a really useful sleep well-being therapy and relaxation aid, especially for anyone suffering from jet lag. Infrared saunas are quite different to traditional saunas as the air is dry and breathable and your body warms up in a beneficial way for your physiology.

There is more to this than just relaxation self-care. Remember the science of your temperature minimum and how this affects jet lag along with your body clock (see page 241)? New evidence published by the National Library of Medicine states that infrared sauna therapy can help with the side effects of chronic fatigue syndrome and help regulate hormones in our body that assist with better-quality sleep.[24] Infrared waves raise your core temperature, your body starts to discharge toxins while the muscles and joints begin to relax and your brain starts releasing melatonin. As your body cools off after a session in an infrared sauna, it sends signals - in the form of more melatonin -

to your brain that it is ready to sleep, which helps send you off into your dreams even faster.

Infrared saunas help your body with thermoregulation and facilitate a parasympathetic state, where the body can more effectively digest and, more importantly, rest.

I find this amazing and, when I can, I try to seek out a sauna session, especially if I'm travelling away with work and need to care for my challenged body clock.

FINANCIAL STRESS

In my work, people frequently open up to me about the impact of financial stress on their sleep health.

The connection between finances and sleep is twofold. The first part of the equation has to do with the stress itself. Financial stress isn't an anomaly. It's a widespread concern for nearly all of us these days.

Within the last few years, money stress has ranked second as the most common source of stress for the average individual.[25] On top of that, the modern fiscal pressure on younger generations has made money matters the number one source of stress for both Gen Z and millennials – and that was before the Covid-19 pandemic added fuel to the fire by crippling the global economy.

'Financial-somnia' describes sleep problems brought on by money-related stressors. Stressors may include losing a job, having poor credit, swimming in what feels like never-ending debt, or something else. Everyone experiences financial stress in their lives, but consistently losing sleep over money-related stress could mean you're struggling with financial-somnia.

To top things off, if you're sleep-deprived, the issue can come full circle. It's been shown that lack of sleep can directly and negatively impact your financial decision-making skills.[26] In other words, if your financial stress disrupts your sleep, the lack of sleep can ultimately cause you to make more bad financial decisions.

ACTION: WHAT IS CREATING YOUR FINANCIAL STRESS?

It's a loaded and likely unpleasant question to ask, but it must be done. If you don't remove the source of your chronic stress first, it will find a way to undermine even the most elaborate sleep-promoting activity. So, start the process of restoring your sleep by identifying your financial stressors:

_____

_____

_____

How the Sleep Reset can help

Learn everything you can about financial health and invest in a really supportive Sleep Reset. This will help soothe your stress and empower you to focus on one thing you can control: your sleep health and well-being.

If you feel that financial stress is the most obvious handbrake on your sleep well-being, really deep dive into Week 4. Understanding more about the sleep–stress connection (see page 143) will give you a cost-free head start in overcoming this sleep hurdle. Prioritising the 'Think in ink' tool (page 98) alongside sleep hypnosis will help you solve your sleep stress at the unconscious level.

I worked with Luke, who had recently bought his first house but on a really unfavourable mortgage rate. Like me in my youth, he had a history of accumulating impulsive debt and had worked really hard to shake off money fear that seemed to haunt him at night. He had been putting off bedtime due to this money stress anxiety, which, when we unpacked it, he saw was an obvious 'self-coping' strategy that was working against his sleep. So we took it slowly. Most of the fear, like all anxiety, was really in his head, and by taking active recovery - disciplined simple gratitude as he hit the pillow, instead of runaway disaster planning - he made huge improvements in his sleep, which helped him create a strong 'power hour' routine to get his money 'house' in order and fuel a better rhythm of well-being throughout his day.

HORMONAL CHANGES FOR WOMEN

I know this section won't be relevant for some of you, but I see so many women suffering each month with disrupted sleep and bouts of hormonal sleep disturbances that I had to write about the impact of the female sleep story when it comes to sleep health.

There are many ways in which women experience sleep differently from men. We biologically respond differently to sleep disorders, sleep deprivation and deficiency, and face particular health outcomes as a result of poor sleep.[27] Women are twice as likely to have insomnia as men and much of this has to do with our hormones.[28]

I work closely supporting communities of women and teenage athletes wanting to learn more and navigate their own Sleep Reset throughout the hormonal milestones in a woman's life, namely puberty and periods, pregnancy, the fourth trimester immediately after birth, midlife and the perimenopause and menopause.[29] This support is massively in demand as studies indicate that, during times of hormonal change, women are at an increased risk of sleep disturbances, poor sleep quality and sleep deprivation, as well as sleep disorders such as OSA, RLS and insomnia.[30]

Hormones impact sleep at every stage of life, which is entirely natural. This is an important area of my work and I am committed to helping women deal with hormone-related sleep turbulence. I feel thankful that, in the last five years, we have seen increasing attention be paid to female health, especially sleep health.

'Periodsomnia': how your period can affect your sleep

The menstrual cycle can be one of the most affecting elements of a good night's rest. A survey conducted by the US National Sleep Foundation found that around 30 per cent of women experience disturbed sleep during their periods, with 23 per cent admitting they struggle to get a full eight hours in the week leading up to their period.[31]

Having a healthy self-awareness and knowing when to support yourself with the Sleep Reset tools during this whole week of disrupted sleep health each month is crucial. Here in the UK, we are collectively seeing this reported as 'periodsomnia' and I think it's great that we are talking about this.[32]

According to the Sleep Health Foundation, seven out of ten women claim their sleep pattern changes before their period, with the most common time frame being three to six days before it starts.[33] Again, this highlights the need for extra sleep support.

Many studies have revealed that women who suffer with PMS have poor sleep quality.[34] The reason for this is thought to be because around this time progesterone levels are lower and, during this phase of the menstrual cycle, research shows that women appear to be more prone to mood disorders such as anxiety and depression, leaving them more vulnerable to sleep problems. That's because many of the same chemicals in the brain that can be disrupted in mood disorders are also involved in regulating sleep.[35]

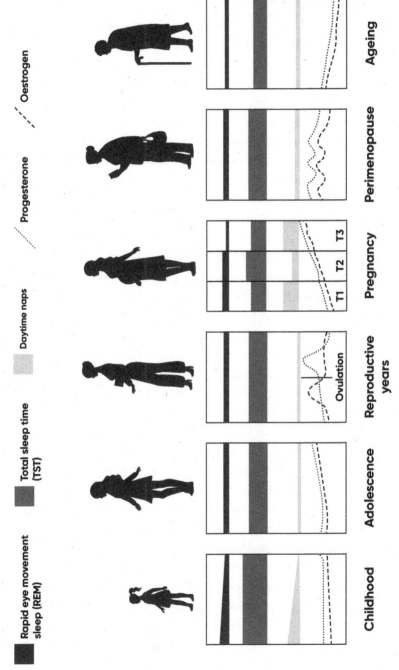

Sleep changes across the female life span

Rapid eye movement sleep (REM) | Total sleep time (TST) | Daytime naps | Progesterone | Oestrogen

Childhood | Adolescence | Reproductive years | Pregnancy | Perimenopause | Ageing

Ovulation

T1 | T2 | T3

*Adapted from Pengo, M.F. et al. 'Sleep in Women Across the Life Span.' Chest 154 (2018): 196–206

Sleep turbulence in pregnancy

I experienced terrible RLS and carpal tunnel syndrome in both my pregnancies and it is often a complete shock if you have always enjoyed good sleep before. Both sleep duration and sleep quality are affected by pregnancy and seem to undergo dynamic changes as the pregnancy progresses. This is why I set up my 'Pimp Your Sleep' workshops to support female sleep in the fourth trimester – the 12 weeks after birth. Just like in this book, the tools in the workshop spoke to the benefits of having a healthy sleep mindset, making use of daytime microbreaks and the importance of mind and body rituals. These moments of hormonal and pregnancy-induced natural sleep challenge are in fact the very best time for you to actively focus on a Sleep Reset.

Balancing menopause symptoms and sleep

The menopause, a natural part of the female midlife life cycle, typically occurs between 40 and 55 years of age as a woman's oestrogen levels decline. It can begin earlier or later and symptoms include hot flushes, chills, weight gain, mood changes and night sweats. Sleep turbulence is often the number one complaint from women who are in the perimenopause (the chapter when your body starts changing hormonally just before you enter menopause) and post-menopause. In fact, the 2005 National Institutes of Health State-of-the-Science Conference Statement cites sleep disturbance as a core symptom of menopause.[36] Among dozens of other symptoms of menopause, hot flushes and night sweats play a major role in sleep disturbances in menopausal women.[37]

Many women in this age bracket also contend with work burnout and family stress, which, as we saw in Week 4, can also interfere with the quality of your sleep.

In my practice, I see many women for the first time when they're experiencing the challenges that the perimenopause brings. The perimenopause can disrupt sleep routines on a regular basis due to its physical, mental and emotional symptoms. Aside from hot flushes, their sleep problems can include difficulty getting to sleep, waking during the night and waking up very early. Over a quarter of women experience sleep problems that really impact daytime functioning and quality of life.[38] Additionally, the most common psychological symptoms, exacerbated by sleep deprivation, are a loss of self-esteem, reduced confidence and heightened anxiety, further highlighting this three-way relationship between sleep, hormones and mood.[39]

I met Jani through my workplace well-being sessions. She was surprised when early perimenopause started to dramatically change her sleep, challenging her work life and sense of self. She hadn't been fully aware of the 40-plus symptoms of the perimenopause and experienced RLS, a racing heart and mind, and long periods of being wide awake during the night.

Choosing to widen the focus away from one night of sleep stress and spend a month focusing on herself gave Jani precious time to embark on her own Sleep Reset, which fuelled a wider, more compassionate lens for all areas of her well-being. She deeply understood that her sleep health powered every aspect of her life and that habit change was easier than she thought. Layering in the audio tools helped her to create a better mindset at work and coached her in the ability to cool down in her mind. Waking at night, Jani decided to learn to 'just chill in my bones', as she put it, rather than toss and turn in a highly active, hot melting pot of frustration and thoughts of *Why me?*, punctuated by hellish future predictions.

Tweaking her caffeine timing, opting for botanical blends and choosing mid-week sobriety instead of her usual nightcap or two gave her back her mental edge and her sleep quality quickly improved. So too did her RLS!

Instead of depriving herself, she curated a strong sleep routine that was sustainable five days a week, relaxing into the weekend while also maintaining her Reset and using a wind-down routine that supported her. She got her family fully on board, paying daily attention to light, dark and movement, and found space to put herself first to sustain her midlife brilliance and build the energy to give back to and care for others. The addition of an evening stroll gave her time to consider her day and she would also visualise this walk just before going to sleep. These small daily changes created a bespoke recovery routine for Jani.

TIPS ON HANDLING SYMPTOMS OF THE PERIMENOPAUSE AND MENOPAUSE

About 75 per cent of menopausal and perimenopausal women battle sudden feelings of heat that can leave night clothes and bedsheets soaked with sweat.[40] These disruptive and uncomfortable vasomotor symptoms, more commonly known as hot flushes and night sweats, are common complaints among midlife women and are intense heat-dissipation responses to small increases in core body temperature, which are caused by a woman's changing hormone levels.

While hormone treatments are highly effective in treating hot flushes during menopause, some easy lifestyle changes can also help you sleep better:

- Make sure the temperature in your bedroom is cool (around 16–18°C is ideal). Try turning down the thermostat before bed.

- Ensure that your room is well ventilated.

- Sleep with a fan on your nightstand.

- Turn your pillow over frequently.

- Invest in natural fibre pillows and mattresses, and bed linens that breathe well, like linen or high-thread-count quality cotton bedsheets rather than synthetic materials (see page 29).

- Wear loose nightclothes and invest in bamboo or breathable cotton sleepwear.

Sleep hypnotherapy is an ideal way to begin coaching your mindset to counterbalance this challenging hormonal health chapter.

For those women who aren't great sleepers to begin with, entering the perimenopause can make insomnia even worse. Hormonal insomnia leaves many women tossing and turning or waking up drenched in sweat. The next day, irritability, anxiety, fatigue and trouble concentrating are not surprisingly commonplace.

How the Sleep Reset can help

The most effective way to support well-being naturally when experiencing hormonal shifts is to learn how to reset your sleep regularly, find the best way to incorporate daily movement (which is further explored in detail in Week 5), especially strength-training, and manage stress through the mind-coaching aspect of the Sleep Reset. The science-supported tools of self-compassion and the potent effects of gratitude are particularly powerful during times of natural hormonal change and challenges (see Week 4). Relearning how to rest and recover if your normal sleeping pattern is disrupted is also crucial to alleviating additional symptoms (see Week 5).

Sleep hypnotherapy is extremely valuable for women's health, especially during the midlife sleep chapters, because hot flushes at night are often cited as one of the most debilitating sleep disrupters. Hypnotherapy has been clinically shown to reduce hot flushes in menopausal women by 80 per cent.[41] These findings reveal that hypnosis can have a direct impact on lessening these occurrences, thereby protecting the valuable emotional well-being sleep we really need during this time of hormonal disturbance.[42]

HEART HEALTH

When you think about keeping your heart healthy, you might imagine high-energy workouts to get it beating faster. But that's not a complete picture of heart health.

The tragic news is that heart disease causes a quarter of all deaths in the UK, with coronary heart disease being the single biggest killer of both men and women worldwide in 2019.[43]

The welcome news is that good sleep is great prevention for heart disease, as we know that sleep and heart health are linked. Heart problems can influence sleep, and sleep can influence heart problems. A fascinating large-scale study, published by the *European Heart Journal* in 2011 and co-authored by Professor Francesco Cappuccio, provides some of the strongest proof yet that sleep duration is a key factor when it comes to heart health.[44]

REGULAR HABITUAL SLEEP IS AT THE CORE OF LOOKING AFTER YOUR HEART HEALTH FOR LIFE.

We know that lack of sleep impacts the cardiovascular system because it's during deep non-REM night-time sleep (see page 87) that, in most people, the body receives the most powerful form of natural blood pressure medication – the heart rate drops and, in turn, blood pressure goes down. In healthy individuals, blood pressure naturally lowers by between 10 and 20 per cent at night, a phenomenon that is sometimes referred to as 'blood pressure dipping'.[45]

Sleep intertwines with other factors that impact cardiovascular health. According to some of the most recent research on sleep and heart health, the heart likes consistent sleep.[46] It's not known why going off a regular sleep schedule (with consistent bed- and wake-up times) affects the heart, but sleep inconsistency may disturb the body's circadian rhythms. Heart rate, blood pressure and other cardiovascular functions vary with the time of day and may become disrupted by inconsistent sleep. Your heart loves good sleep, especially regular sleep and wake-up times. According to a 2022 study in the *European Society of Cardiology*, regardless of chronotype, it appeared that an approximate bedtime of between 10 and 11pm is optimal.[47]

A recent article published in the journal *Hypertension* examined the links between poor sleep and hypertension.[48] It showed that short sleep duration, working a night shift and OSA (see page 222) are all associated with risk for hypertension.

How the Sleep Reset can help

Maintaining an optimum amount of sleep is crucially protective of our cardiovascular systems, blood pressure and overall heart health. Sometimes it's in your best interest to rest (see Week 5). By the same token, a healthy diet, regular exercise and low stress – all outlined in the Sleep Reset – may promote the sort of deep, restorative sleep that is essential for good cardiovascular health.

When you improve sleep, you may see an improvement in blood pressure. Many patients have even been able to decrease or discontinue their medications by working through a Sleep Reset and getting healthier.

SLEEP HEALTH AND CANCER SUPPORT

It's very often the case that, without therapeutic sleep support, people living with a cancer diagnosis will suffer from sleep difficulties, insomnia and circadian misalignment, especially before, during and after treatment. In fact, shockingly it is thought that about 50 per cent of cancer patients will struggle with sleep, with between 30 and 60 per cent experiencing insomnia during their cancer care phases.[49]

Sleep problems may be caused by many factors on top of anxiety and emotional stress, such as the side effects of treatment, medicines and long hospital stays. Cancer can provoke fatigue, sleep disturbances and emotional distress too.

How the Sleep Reset can help

Suffering during this stressful time can be relieved by focusing on sleep well-being and having a Sleep Reset. Many studies have shown that relaxation, sleep hypnosis and behavioural sleep interventions can be incredibly helpful during this time of life and help reduce the trauma impact.[50]

The Sleep Reset is here to help, and I recommend that you engage with the mind–body tools as well as talking with your healthcare team about sleep problems and advocating to protect your precious sleep.

You can consider asking these questions:

- What holistic support for my sleep is on offer?
- Can you recommend a sleep therapist who could help with the problems I am having?
- Ask about any steroids and targeted cancer drugs that can sometimes create sleep challenges and or cause insomnia.
- Timing of the drugs can help. It can help if you take them in the morning, so ask your medical team about this and any other helpful guidance.

Remember that sleep challenges and insomnia are highly treatable and many new sleep research studies have shown that sleep hypnosis and mind–body relaxation have a lasting impact on supporting sleep health in the midst of the cancer journey.[51] One study showed that sleep hypnosis created significant decreases in fatigue, sleep difficulties and emotional distress.[52] Most of these positive effects were maintained at one-year follow-up.

Self-hypnosis shows promising evidence for the self-management of pain and pain-related sleep problems among cancer survivors. In one study, a four-week recorded audio hypnosis intervention helped reduce pain and improve sleep even more than a recorded relaxation intervention in cancer survivors with chronic pain. Both hypnosis and relaxation provided significant and moderate-to-large improvements in pain sleep interference and cancer stress and anxiety at night.[53]

When journalist and author Karen was diagnosed with stage 2 breast cancer, her life and sleep patterns were turned upside down. Chemically induced by chemotherapy drugs into menopause at 43, she was dealing not only with night sweats and insomnia that so often accompany perimenopause and menopause, but also the ravaging side effects of chemotherapy and radiotherapy. This is her story in her own words:

'Following my cancer diagnosis, my sleep health hit rock bottom and I would find myself awake randomly in the middle of the night, sweating, overthinking and with a racing mind about what lay ahead for me. I was also suffering from the discomfort of two operations, the side effects of powerful IV chemo drugs and uncomfortable "scorch" mark burns from the targeted radiotherapy.

'I knew that rest, light exercise, fresh air and daylight were my recovery-based "allies" and would not only improve my sleep but also lead me back to a healthy physical body. I consulted a nutritionist and completely changed my diet. I took gentle exercise - a walk with my dogs, a gentle jog or a sea swim – whenever I felt up to it. I silenced the perfectionist inner voice which had always driven me and allowed myself to rest and take a nap whenever my body needed it. Afternoons were often when I felt at my most tired. When my treatment ended, I slowly but steadily increased my exercise regime to build back up to my pre-illness days. I have largely stayed with the nutrition plan and, 11 years on from my diagnosis, I have never felt better.'

CONCLUSION: CONSOLIDATING THE SLEEP RESET

Well done on all your hard work over the last five weeks! You have achieved so much, demonstrated resilience and shown up for your sleep health in many beneficial ways.

You have seen how small but mighty shifts in your environment and the science of light and dark can help you create the best conditions for healthy sleep. You've also learned about the vital roles that self-compassion and gratitude play in combating sleep stress. You now know how to harness your mindset, access rest and recovery and use movement and nutrition to support your sleep. I know you won't forget the impact of your choices, energy and new-found compassionate focus.

Take a moment now to look back at your Sleep Reset motivation (page 27). What can you celebrate from your journey? There's no doubt that your relationship to sleep has been enhanced. Have you moved closer now to the solutions to your sleep challenge that you were seeking at the start of this book? What would you update?

I'VE GIVEN YOU THE ROAD MAP, BUT YOU'VE DONE THE WORK.

Like other areas of our health, we can think of our sleep in a preventative way rather than only seeking help when sleep feels in crisis. Your sleep needs regular care and attention and, as a therapist and performance coach, I implore you to take this forward and share your sleep health knowledge far and wide.

I can't promise your sleep will always be perfect, but you now have a bespoke set of mindset, breathwork and hypnosis tools to help you improve your sleep and cope with any setbacks along the way.

ACTION: UPDATE YOUR SLEEP RESET COMMITMENT

Take a look back at your Sleep Reset commitment on page 36. Is there anything you now want to change? Define for yourself right now what you will and won't do moving forward by answering the following questions:

- How will you manage your internal voice?

- In what ways will you try to use self-compassion to cope with tricky times?

- What boundaries will you set in your life? (This could be in terms of demands from others, your schedule or your daily nutrition.)

- How will you make rest a part of your daily routine?

- What forms of movement will you think about using?

- What could your nightly wind-down routine look like?

- What sleep-promoting foods will you incorporate into your diet?

Think about all you have learned. What has sparked for you?
What tools will you take with you?

_____

_____

Over the last five weeks, you have had the opportunity to experience everyday ways to fuel better energy, mindset and, of course, protect and look after your all-important sleep health. Regardless of whether you went all-in and worked methodically through the Reset week by week or you chose a focus week to give yourself a simple Sleep Reset, there is one thing that's universal – you'll have taken a giant leap forward in your best rested self.

For lasting improvement, please make the advice in this book a part of your overall lifestyle. Your energy and life are too precious not to. After all, sleep is one-third of your life, and I get to see first hand how small steps and behaviour changes can really energise any sleep stress or struggle. My hope is that all the tools and techniques will support you no matter what challenges you in life. There is no failure here, only temporary setbacks that you can now overcome.

If there's one thing you can take away from this book, it's knowing you can create a sleep health strategy to come back to, time and time again. You can either return to the full Reset any time your sleep needs an MOT or, like any personal well-being strategy, you can build your favourite habits and audio tools into your daily recovery and evening sleep rituals. The choice is yours. The Reset will work whenever you feel your sleep is stressed or needs rescuing from our hyperpaced world of never-ending scrolling. You can rest safe in the confidence that you can now tackle any sleep speed bumps along the way.

COMMIT NOW TO NOT GIVING UP ON YOUR
SLEEP CARE – EVEN ONE OR TWO TOOLS A
DAY PLUS SEEKING MORNING LIGHT CAN
MAKE ALL THE DIFFERENCE.

You've enhanced your relationship to your sleep health and you've found your own sleep solution. Now you can move forward, keeping in mind the following principles that will help to future-proof your sleep health:

Sleep trust: Trust in your body's own sleep system and let it work for you! Your mind and body can self-regulate with your guidance. Realising that short, consolidated sleep often feels more satisfying than longer, fragmented sleep should have helped you develop this trust.

No judgement: It's natural to automatically judge yourself and feel frustrated at being awake in the early hours! But, as we've seen, sleep stress puts a handbrake on the natural process of sleep, so choose to leave it behind.

Acceptance: Choosing to acknowledge your natural capacity for change while also adopting a friendly, consistent approach to sleep health is an important step for sleep today, tomorrow and for life.

Patience: It is unlikely that both the quality and quantity of your sleep were optimal straightaway after just one night, but the steps in this book have both supported your sleep health and anchored in a healthy, friendly and informed approach that you are now on board with and can take forward to future-proof your sleep.

I'm excited about your progress, for this is just the beginning. By reading this book, you have decided to put sleep health at the front and centre of your well-being. Remember that your journey to better sleep started the moment you chose to embrace sleep as your superpower for living a full and healthy life.

As you now know, sleep starts from the moment you wake up. Looking after your future sleep is now in your capable hands!

KNOWING HOW TO LOOK AFTER YOUR SLEEP HEALTH IS THE SPRINGBOARD FOR GREATER EVERYDAY WELLNESS TODAY, TONIGHT, FOR LIFE.

ACKNOWLEDGEMENTS

There simply would be no book, no method, without the real sleep stories and everyday courage of all of the hard-working, stressed, tired, curious minds and all the brilliant people who have allowed me to pitch a seat up by their side, listen to them and coach them. Together we have created this realistic, life-changing approach.

To everyone who called in to live radio, listened to my talks, stayed back to debate behaviour change and to all of the brilliant students and sceptics who believed in change and stayed with the process, every single one of you continues to inspire me, each and every week.

Enormous gratitude to the most stunningly wise talent that is my editor and guide, Julia Kellaway, and to the visionary Sam Jackson for her unwavering belief in my ability to share this essential sleep support. And to my team, especially Valeria Huerta, for making the dream come true.

To my home team, my very own fab four: my co-pilot and life partner, Paul; my greatest teachers, Darcy and Jude; and, of course, the original nap boss, my golden retriever, Honey. You celebrated every part of me while bringing the gifts of humour, space and time. Through the plot twists of the pandemic and personal surgery, you gave me all the energy and resilience I needed to eventually bring this book to life.

Thanks to all the brilliant researchers, leaders, change-makers and athletes who have allowed me to be their performance well-being coach and to all the career mentors and partnerships that have helped shaped how I teach: the outstanding mentor that is Mike Weeks and his colleague Professor Ian Snape at Frontline Mind; Professor Chris Idzikowski; Dr Patrizia Collard; sport sleep coach Nick Littlehales for being a fellow change-maker helping to put sleep first in sport; fellow hypnotherapists in my field, Marcia Tilman and Lynda Hudson; Gemma Evans, founder of Health Hackers; James Keen and the team at Hypnos Beds for your visionary understanding of sleep well-being so many years ago; the outstanding sleep community that is the British Sleep Society, the European Sleep Research Society and the Royal Society of Medicine for all the continuous research insight and CPD and for setting me on this continuous pathway to forever learning; to those across the Atlantic whose work has always fascinated me: Dr Shauna Shapiro, Dr Alia Crum, Dr David Spiegel and Dr Andrew Huberman; of course, here in the UK, all the brilliant NHS consultants who changed my life with your mind–body holistic understanding and all the hard-working GPs, especially the brilliant GP (for over 22 years and counting), my colleague and lifestyle medicine friend, Dr Hamendra Patel, who trusted me to share my sleep health method within the wider community and change lives forever through the power of sleep.

RESOURCES

I am often asked how I support my own rest and recovery. Here are some further tools I find beneficial.

Mindtonicsleep.com (Sleep Reset Hub)
My own website has a dedicated Sleep Reset section containing some helpful worksheets, the audio tools and some of the transcripts to support your sleep health journey. It is jam-packed with case studies and helpful insight that may be useful for your sleep well-being.

WIDER SLEEP HEALTH SUPPORT

There are so many sleep disorders and, depending on your own struggles, I encourage you to explore your local sleep support services and chat to your GP and health providers. The two charities below also have some excellent resources.

Hope2Sleep
https://www.hope2sleep.co.uk/
Set up by the amazing Kath Hope, this is a unique charity that supports patients with all kinds of sleep disordered breathing.

The Sleep Charity
https://thesleepcharity.org.uk/
This charity runs a brilliant national sleep helpline in the UK: 03303 530 541.

FURTHER READING

The Anxiety Solution by Chloe Brotheridge (Michael Joseph, 2017)
Chloe's work is inspiring and I share it in all my teen sleep roadshows.

Breath by James Nestor (Penguin Life, 2021)
The most fascinating introduction to the inner magic of your breath.

Flow by Mihaly Csikszentmihalyi (Rider, 2002)
The classic work that inspired my fascination with meaningful energy.

How to Overcome Trauma and Find Yourself Again by Dr Jessamy Hibberd (Aster, 2023)
A brilliant book sharing insight on how to overcome inner turmoil and adapt to life's plot twists. I am a personal fan of her work and all her books. Essential reading to help you lay your head on the pillow in peace.

Power Hour by Adrienne Herbert (Penguin, 2022)
I love Adrienne and her incredible book and podcast. Not only is she a great friend, but this relatable, inspiring book gets you out of the starting gate into morning action.

Resilience By Design by Mike Weeks and Ian Snape (Wiley, 2021)
The definitive guide to resilience for everyone who wants to reach their full potential.

Rest by Alex Soojung-Kim Pang (Penguin Life, 2018)
I have championed this visionary approach to the power of rest in every project I lead.

Rest Is Resistance by Tricia Hersey (Aster, 2022)
This book stopped me in my tracks – I love Tricia's unwavering belief that we must reclaim our rest, and how rest can provide deep healing.

Self Compassion by Kristin Neff (Yellow Kite, 2011)
In my biggest sleep and parenting challenges, Dr Neff illuminated the power of kindness to create behaviour change in me forever.

The Circadian Code by Dr Satchin Panda (Vermilion, 2018)
Dr Panda's lab work has been game-changing for the field of sleep health and understanding that when we eat is just as influential as how we eat for wider health.

The Mindfulness Bible by Dr Patrizia Collard (Godsfield Press, 2015)
This comprehensive book, written by a mentor of mine, explores the history of mindfulness, presents the key pioneers and brilliantly charts the way in which mindfulness is applied in Western psychology and therapy. I always recommend this book for those who want to explore mindfulness further.

The Self-Care Cookbook by Gemma Ogston (Vermilion, 2019)
As a massive foodie, I love Gemma's approach that food is to nourish and bring us joy but also plays a part in fuelling our self-care. She has delicious, nutritious recipes and I love her exciting plant-based approach.

The Wim Hof Method by Wim Hof (Rider, 2022)
Wim Hof's powerful story and definitive guide cannot fail to light the fire of discovering your human potential. He has really transformed many lives through his brilliant dedication to helping us reach our true potential.

Why We Sleep by Matthew Walker (Penguin, 2018)
This world-class, relatable sleep science book is a must-read if you are as passionate about one-third of your life as I am.

The following fellow experts changed my life through their work and dedication to unravelling the mind–body connection with relatable expert guidance and insight:

- *Eat More Live Well*, Dr Megan Rossi (Penguin Life, 2021)
- *Food for Life*, Tim Spector (Jonathan Cape, 2022)
- *How to Build a Healthy Brain*, Kimberley Wilson (Yellow Kite, 2022)
- *How to Go Plant-Based*, Ella Mills (Yellow Kite, 2022)
- *The Beautiful Cure*, Daniel M. Davis (Vintage, 2019)
- *The Body Keeps the Score*, Bessel van der Kolk (Penguin, 2015)
- *When the Body Says No* (Vermilion, 2019) and *Scattered Minds* (Vermilion, 2019), Gabor Maté

MY SLEEP HEALTH RECOMMENDATIONS

Beds
Hypnos beds and mattresses
www.hypnosbeds.com
I've been working with Hypnos for over five years and it is the brand I endorse. They provide the highest levels of quality and comfort while pioneering sustainable and ethical bed-making.

Blue-light screen filters
Ocushield
www.ocushield.com
Designed by optometrists and recommended by sleep experts, this range of blue-light screen protectors and glasses filter out harmful blue light to protect your sleep health, eyes and skin, and I'm a huge fan!

Earplugs/earphones
Flare Audio
www.flareaudio.com
A small in-ear device that reduces trigger noises for a peaceful night's sleep.

Jet lag

British Airways jet lag tool

www.britishairways.com/travel/drsleep/

One of my mentors and sleep science friends, Professor Chris Idzikowski, designed this free BA jet lag tool and it's great!

Light therapy

Lumie light

www.lumie.com

Lumie is a member of the Society for Light Treatment and Biological Rhythms (SLTBR), an international group devoted to promoting research and knowledge about the biological effects of light. I love my Wake-up and Vitamin L Lumie lights and use them both for keeping track of healthy light/dark levels for energy and sleep.

Philips Hue

www.philips-hue.com

I especially love the Philips Hue Go lights and bulbs and my teens are big fans of the portable colour-changing light, which is ideal for cosy, sleep-protecting red light at night. I really rate this when working with families for child and teen sleep.

Selfie light

Available from many online retailers, this is a great low-cost option for helping with SAD, morning alertness or daytime energy.

Nutrition

Bare Biology

www.barebiology.com

When it comes to omega-3 supplements, I personally rate this family-owned, UK company that makes the best possible supplements from Norwegian and European ingredients, with complete transparency so you know exactly what you're taking.

BetterYou

www.betteryou.com

I use their pill-free, bioavailable vitamin sprays and transdermal magnesium lotions for a peaceful night's sleep.

Chuckling Goat

www.chucklinggoat.co.uk

I use their Original Kefir daily for my morning shot of happy sleep–gut health.

Deliciously Ella

www.deliciouslyella.com

I am ever thankful to Ella Mills and the Deliciously Ella team for fuelling my sleep health with her visionary recipes and community.

DIRTEA

www.dirteaworld.com

This is the UK brand I choose for their great-tasting, safe and very high-quality reishi mushroom powder, which is naturally caffeine free and 100 per cent organic.

Form

www.formnutrition.com

I use their plant-based, sleep-friendly protein powder every day, and it tastes amazing with just water!

KLORIS

www.kloriscbd.com/pages/cbd-for-sleep

A female-founded British wellness brand that creates superior-grade, sustainably made, broad-spectrum, organic CBD oils and skincare, formulated by plant scientists.

Leapfrog Remedies

www.leapfrogremedies.com

I love to champion this brand's 'Snooze' range as it's packed with sleep hero ingredients lactium and lactoferrin. My neurodivergent teens love the berry taste and it massively helps them wind down.

Lumity

www.lumitylife.co.uk

Founded by the brilliant biologist Dr Sara Palmer, this science-powered range of supplements to support circadian health and nighttime wellness is my go-to choice. The 'Morning & Night' range is high quality and packed with sleep support nutrients.

Teapigs

www.teapigs.co.uk

I am a fan of their matcha chai latte sachets.

Sleep apnoea

Acurable

acurable.com

The AcuPebble SA1000 is a brilliant, patient-friendly wearable medical device for home sleep apnoea testing.

Philips Respironics

www.philips.co.uk/healthcare/solutions/sleep-and-respiratory-care

Philips makes incredible sleep apnoea products, great for supportive sleep health at home.

Vagus nerve toning

Sensate

www.getsensate.com

A groundbreaking innovation in wellness technology, Sensate uses the natural power of sonic resonance to calm your body's nervous system, providing immediate relief and long-term benefits from regular use. This is a genius sleep tech device that I personally love for my sleep health!

Weighted blankets

Aeyla

www.aeyla.co.uk

In our neurodiverse family, these are favourites. Most notably, the Dreamer blanket helps keep a sleep-friendly temperature and feels like a giant, restful, calming hug.

REFERENCES

Introduction

1. Peng, J., Zhang, T., Li, Y., Wu, L., Peng, X., Li, C., Lin, X., Yu, J., Mao, L., Sun, J., Fang, P., 'Effects of dysfunctional beliefs about sleep on sleep quality and mental health among patients with *COVID*-19 treated in Fangcang shelter hospitals.' *Frontiers in Public Health* 11 (2023) doi: 10.3389/fpubh.2023.1129322

   Li, Y., Sahakian, B.J., et al., 'The brain structure and genetic mechanisms underlying the nonlinear association between sleep duration, cognition and mental health.' *Nature Aging* 2 (2022): 425–37. doi: 10.1038/s43587-022-00210-2

   Watson, N.F., Badr, M.S., Belenky, G., Bliwise, D.L., Buxton, O.M., Buysse, D., Dinges, D.F., Gangwisch, J., Grandner, M.A., Kushida, C., Malhotra, R.K., Martin, J.L., Patel, S.R., Quan, S.F., Tasali, E., 'Recommended Amount of Sleep for a Healthy Adult: A Joint Consensus Statement of the American Academy of Sleep Medicine and Sleep Research Society.' *Sleep* 38, 6 (2015): 843–4. doi: 10.5665/sleep.4716

   Edinger, J.D., Wohlgemuth, W.K., Radtke, R.A., Marsh, G.R., Quillian, R.E. 'Does cognitive-behavioral insomnia therapy alter dysfunctional beliefs about sleep?' *Sleep* 24, 5 (2001): 591–9. doi: 10.1093/sleep/24.5.591

   Morin, C.M., Vallières, A., Ivers, H., 'Dysfunctional beliefs and attitudes about sleep (*DBAS*): validation of a brief version (*DBAS*-16)' *Sleep* 30, 11 (2007): 1547–54. doi: 10.1093/sleep/30.11.1547

2. Blume, C., Garbazza, C., Spitschan, M., 'Effects of light on human circadian rhythms, sleep and mood.' *Somnologie (Berl)* 23, 3 (2019): 147–156. doi: 10.1007/s11818-019-00215-x

   Lucas, R.J., Lall, G.S., Allen, A.E., Brown, T.M. 'How rod, cone, and melanopsin photoreceptors come together to enlighten the mammalian circadian clock.' *Progress in Brain Research* 199 (2012): 1–18. doi: 10.1016/b978-0-444-59427-3.00001-0

   Lockley, S.W., Evans, E.E., Scheer, F.A.J.L., Brainard, G.C., Czeisler, C.A., Aeschbach, D., 'Short-wavelength sensitivity for the direct effects of light on alertness, vigilance, and the waking electroencephalogram in humans.' *Sleep* 29, 2 (2006): 161–8.

Siraji, M.A., Kalavally, V., Schaefer, A., Haque, S. 'Effects of Daytime Electric Light Exposure on Human Alertness and Higher Cognitive Functions: A Systematic Review.' *Frontiers in Psychology* 12 (2022). doi: 10.3389/fpsyg.2021.765750

Walker, W.H., Walton, J.C., DeVries, A.C., et al. 'Circadian rhythm disruption and mental health.' *Translational Psychiatry* 10, 28 (2020). https://doi.org/10.1038/s41398-020-0694-0

3. Butz S., Stahlberg D., 'The Relationship between Self-Compassion and Sleep Quality: An Overview of a Seven-Year German Research Program.' *Behavioral Sciences (Basel)* 10, 3 (2020): 64. doi: 10.3390/bs10030064

4. Kalmbach, D.A., Anderson, J.R., Drake, C.L., 'The impact of stress on sleep: Pathogenic sleep reactivity as a vulnerability to insomnia and circadian disorders.' *Journal of Sleep Research* 27, 6 (2018). doi: 10.1111/jsr.12710

'Sleep-deprived and anxious? This brain region helps to explain why.' *Nature* 575, 261 (2019). doi: https://doi.org/10.1038/d41586-019-03380-z

Palagini, L., Hertenstein, E., Riemann, D., Nissen, C., 'Sleep, insomnia and mental health.' *Journal of Sleep Research* 31, 4 (2022). doi: 10.1111/jsr.13628

5. Laborde, S., Hosang, T., Mosley, E., Dosseville, F., 'Influence of a 30-Day Slow-Paced Breathing Intervention Compared to Social Media Use on Subjective Sleep Quality and Cardiac Vagal Activity.' *Journal of Clinical Medicine* 8, 2 (2019): 193. doi: 10.3390/jcm8020193

6. Lavie, P., 'Insomnia and sleep-disordered breathing', *Sleep Medicine* 8, 4 (2007): S21–25. doi.org/10.1016/s1389-9457(08)70005-4

Janssen, H.C.J.P., Venekamp, L.N., Peeters, G.A.M., Pijpers, A., Pevernagie, D.A.A., 'Management of insomnia in sleep disordered breathing.' *European Respiratory Review* 28, 153 (2019). doi: 10.1183/16000617.0080-2019

7. Besedovsky, L., Cordi, M., Wißlicen, L., et al., 'Hypnotic enhancement of slow-wave sleep increases sleep-associated hormone secretion and reduces sympathetic predominance in healthy humans.' *Communications Biology* 5, 747 (2022). https://doi.org/10.1038/s42003-022-03643-y

Chamine, I., Atchley, R., Oken, B.S., 'Hypnosis Intervention Effects on Sleep Outcomes: A Systematic Review.' *Journal of Clinical Sleep Medicine* 14, 2 (2018): 271–283. doi: 10.5664/jcsm.6952

Cordi, M.J., Schlarb, A.A., Rasch, B., 'Deepening sleep by hypnotic suggestion.' *Sleep* 37, 6 (2014):1143–52, 1152A–1152F. doi: 10.5665/sleep.3778

Thompson, T., Terhune, D.B., Oram, C., Sharangparni, J., Rouf, R., Solmi, M., Veronese, N., Stubbs, B., 'The effectiveness of hypnosis for pain relief: A systematic review and meta-analysis of 85 controlled experimental trials.' *Neuroscience & Biobehavioral Reviews* 99 (2019): 298–310. doi: 10.1016/j.neubiorev.2019.02.013

8. Jiang, H., White, M.P., Greicius, M.D., Waelde, L.C., Spiegel, D. 'Brain Activity and Functional Connectivity Associated with Hypnosis', *Cerebral Cortex* 27, 8 (2017): 4083–93. doi: 10.1093/cercor/bhw220

Kittle, J., Spiegel, D., 'Hypnosis: The Most Effective Treatment You Have Yet to Prescribe.' *American Journal of Medicine* 134, 3 (2021): 304–5. doi: 10.1016/j.amjmed.2020.10.010

9. Gruzelier, J.H., 'A Review of the Impact of Hypnosis, Relaxation, Guided Imagery and Individual Differences on Aspects of Immunity and Health.' *Stress* 5, 2 (2002): 147–63. doi: 10.1080/10253890290027877

Lam, T.H., Chung, K.F., Yeung, W.F., Yu, B.Y., Yung, K.P., Ng, T.H., 'Hypnotherapy for insomnia: a systematic review and meta-analysis of randomized controlled trials.' *Complementary Therapies in Medicine* 23, 5 (2015): 719–32. doi: 10.1016/j.ctim.2015.07.011

Tuominen, J., Kallio, S., Kaasinen, V., Railo, H., 'Segregated brain state during hypnosis.' *Neuroscience of Consciousness* 2021, 1 (2021). https://doi.org/10.1093/nc/niab002

10. Black, D.S., O'Reilly, G.A., Olmstead, R., Breen, E.C., Irwin, M.R., 'Mindfulness meditation and improvement in sleep quality and daytime impairment among older adults with sleep disturbances: a randomized clinical trial.' *JAMA Internal Medicine* 175, 4 (2015): 494–501. doi: 10.1001/jamainternmed.2014.8081

Lau, W.K.W., Leung, M.K., Wing, Y.K., et al., 'Potential Mechanisms of Mindfulness in Improving Sleep and Distress.' *Mindfulness* 9 (2018): 547–555. https://doi.org/10.1007/s12671-017-0796-9

Peters, A.L., Saunders, W.J., Jackson, M.L. 'Mindfulness-Based Strategies for Improving Sleep in People with Psychiatric Disorders.' *Current Psychiatry Reports* 24 (2022): 645–60. https://doi.org/10.1007/s11920-022-01370-z

Before We Begin

1. Walker, M.P., Stickgold, R., 'Sleep, memory, and plasticity.' *Annual Review of Psychology* 57 (2006): 139–66. doi: 10.1146/annurev.psych.56.091103.070307

Xie, L., Kang, H., Xu, Q., Chen, M.J., Liao, Y., Thiyagarajan, M., O'Donnell, J., Christensen, D.J., Nicholson, C., Iliff, J.J., Takano, T., Deane, R., Nedergaard, M., 'Sleep drives metabolite clearance from the adult brain.' *Science* 342, 6156 (2013): 373–7. doi: 10.1126/science

2. Robbins, R., Grandner, M.A., Buxton, O.M, Hale, L, Buysse, D.J., Knutson, K.L., Patel, S.R., Troxel, W.M., Youngstedt, S.D., Czeisler, C.A., Jean-Louis, G., 'Sleep myths: an expert-led study to identify false beliefs about sleep that impinge upon population sleep health practices.' *Sleep Health*, 5, 4 (2019). https://doi.org/10.1016/j.sleh.2019.02.002

Dinges, D.F., Pack, F., Williams, K., Gillen, K.A., Powell, J.W., Ott, G.E., Aptowicz, C., Pack, A.I., 'Cumulative sleepiness, mood disturbance, and psychomotor vigilance performance decrements during a week of sleep restricted to 4–5 hours per night.' *Sleep* 20, 4 (1997): 267–77. PMID: 9231952

Shi, G., Xing, L., Wu, D., Bhattacharyya, B.J., Jones, C.R., McMahon, T., Chong, S.Y.C., Chen, J.A., Coppola, G., Geschwind, D., Krystal, A., Ptáček, L.J., Fu, Y.H., 'A Rare Mutation of β1-Adrenergic Receptor Affects Sleep/Wake Behaviors.' *Neuron* 103, 6 (2019):1044–55 doi: 10.1016/j.neuron.2019.07.026

3. Prather, A.A., Pressman, S.D., Miller, G.E., et al., 'Temporal Links Between Self-Reported Sleep and Antibody Responses to the Influenza Vaccine.' *International Journal of Behavioral Medicine* 28 (2021): 151–8. https://doi.org/10.1007/s12529-020-09879-4

Besedovsky, L., Lange, T. and Haack, M., 'The Sleep-Immune Crosstalk in Health and Disease.' *Physiological Reviews* 99, 3 (2019): 1325–80.

4. Knowles, O.E, Drinkwater, E.J., Urwin, C.S., Lamon, S., Aisbett, B., 'Inadequate sleep and muscle strength: Implications for resistance training.' *Journal of Science and Medicine in Sport* 21, 9 (2018): 959–68. doi: 10.1016/j.jsams.2018.01.012

Chen, Y., Cui, Y., Chen, S., Wu, Z., 'Relationship between sleep and muscle strength among Chinese university students: a cross-sectional study.' *Journal of Musculoskeletal and Neuronal Interactions* 17, 4 (2017): 327–33.

5. Sharma, S., Kavuru, M., 'Sleep and metabolism: an overview.' *International Journal of Endocrinology* (2010). doi: 10.1155/2010/270832

6. Bigalke, J.A., Shan, Z., Carter, J.R., 'Orexin, Sleep, Sympathetic Neural Activity, and Cardiovascular Function.' *Hypertension* 79, 12 (2022): 2643–55. doi: 10.1161/*HYPERTENSIONAHA*.122.19796

7. Stranges, S., Tigbe, W., Gómez-Olivé, F.X., Thorogood, M., Kandala, N.B., 'Sleep problems: an emerging global epidemic? Findings from the *INDEPTH WHO-SAGE* study among more than 40,000 older adults from 8 countries across Africa and Asia.' *Sleep* 35, 8 (2012): 1173–81. doi: 10.5665/sleep.2012

Bhaskar, S., Hemavathy, D., Prasad, S., 'Prevalence of chronic insomnia in adult patients and its correlation with medical comorbidities.' *Journal of Family Medicine and Primary Care* 5, 4 (2016): 780–4. doi: 10.4103/2249-4863.201153

'The Global Pursuit of Better Sleep Health.' *Philips* (2019), https://www.philips.com/c-dam/b2c/master/experience/smartsleep/world-sleep-day/2019/2019-philips-world-sleep-day-survey-results.pdf?_ga=2.202020051.319545962.1697646065-1140880154.1697646065

8. Miner, B., Kryger, M.H., 'Sleep in the Aging Population.' *Sleep Medicine Clinics* 12, 1 (2017): 31–8. doi: 10.1016/j.jsmc.2016.10.008

Tatineny, P., Shafi, F., Gohar, A., Bhat, A., 'Sleep in the Elderly.' *Missouri Medicine* 117, 5 (2020): 490–5.

9. Ancoli-Israel, S., Bliwise, D.L., Nørgaard,J.P., 'The effect of nocturia on sleep.' *Sleep Medicine Reviews* 15, 2 (2011). https://doi.org/10.1016/j.smrv.2010. 03.002

   Weiss, J.P., 'Nocturia: focus on etiology and consequences.' *Reviews in Urology* 14, 3–4 (2012): 48–55

   Tikkinen, K. A., Tammela, T. L., Huhtala, H., Auvinen, A., 'Is nocturia equally common among men and women? A population based study in Finland.' *The Journal of Urology* 175, 2 (2006): 596–600. https://doi.org/10.1016/s0022-5347(05)00245-4

10. Jehan, S., Masters-Isarilov, A., Salifu, I., Zizi, F., Jean-Louis, G., Pandi-Perumal, S.R., Gupta, R., Brzezinski, A., McFarlane, S.I., 'Sleep Disorders in Postmenopausal Women.' *Journal of Sleep Disorders & Therapy* 4, 5 (2015): 212.

    Guidozzi F., 'Sleep and sleep disorders in menopausal women.' *Climacteric* 16, 2 (2013): 214–19. doi: 10.3109/13697137.2012.753873

    Walsleben, J.A., 'Women and sleep.' *Handbook of Clinical Neurology* 98 (2011): 639–51. doi: 10.1016/B978-0-444-52006-7.00040-X. *PMID*: 21056215

11. Lechner, M., Breeze, C.E., Ohayon, M.M., Kotecha, B. 'Snoring and breathing pauses during sleep: interview survey of a United Kingdom population sample reveals a significant increase in the rates of sleep apnoea and obesity over the last 20 years – data from the UK sleep survey.' *Sleep Medicine* 54 (2019): 250–6. doi: 10.1016/j.sleep.2018.08.029. Epub 2018 Oct 9. PMID: 30597439

    Benjafield, A.V., Ayas, N.T., Eastwood, P.R., Heinzer, R., Ip, M.S.M., Morrell, M.J., Nunez, C.M., Patel, S.R., Penzel, T., Pépin, J.L., Peppard, P.E., Sinha, S., Tufik, S., Valentine, K., Malhotra, A., 'Estimation of the global prevalence and burden of obstructive sleep apnoea: a literature-based analysis.' Lancet Respiratory Medicine 7, 8 (2019): 687–98. doi: 10.1016/S2213-2600(19)30198-5

    'Sleep apnoea.' *NHS UK*, www.nhs.uk/conditions/sleep-apnoea/

12. Becker, P.M., 'The biopsychosocial effects of restless legs syndrome (RLS).' *Neuropsychiatric Disease and Treatment* 2, 4 (2006): 505–12. doi: 10.2147/nedt. 2006.2.4.505

13. Okamoto-Mizuno, K., Mizuno, K., 'Effects of thermal environment on sleep and circadian rhythm.' *Journal of Physiological Anthropology* 31, 14 (2012). https://doi.org/10.1186/1880-6805-31-14

    Obradovich, N., Migliorini, R., Mednick, S.C., Fowler, J.H., 'Nighttime temperature and human sleep loss in a changing climate.' *Science Advances* 3, 5 (2017). doi: 10.1126/sciadv.1601555

Murphy, P.J., Campbell, S.S., 'Nighttime drop in body temperature: a physiological trigger for sleep onset?' *Sleep* 20, 7 (1997): 505–11. doi: 10.1093/sleep/20.7.505

14. Grinde, B., Patil, G.G., 'Biophilia: does visual contact with nature impact on health and well-being?' *International Journal of Environmental Research and Public Health* 6, 9 (2009): 2332–43. doi: 10.3390/ijerph6092332

Jimenez, M.P., DeVille, N.V., Elliott, E.G., Schiff, J.E., Wilt, G.E., Hart, J.E., James, P., 'Associations between Nature Exposure and Health: A Review of the Evidence.' *International Journal of Environmental Research and Public Health*, 18, 9 (2021): 4790. doi: 10.3390/ijerph18094790

Huntsman, D.D., Bulaj, G., 'Healthy Dwelling: Design of Biophilic Interior Environments Fostering Self-Care Practices for People Living with Migraines, Chronic Pain, and Depression.' *International Journal of Environmental Research and Public Health* 19, 4 (2022): 2248. doi: 10.3390/ijerph19042248

15. Fan, X., Liao, C., Bivolarova, M.P., Sekhar, C., Laverge, J., Lan, L., Mainka, A., Akimoto, M., Wargocki, P., 'A field intervention study of the effects of window and door opening on bedroom *IAQ*, sleep quality, and next-day cognitive performance.' *Building and Environment* 225 (2022). https://doi.org/10.1016/j.buildenv.2022.109630

Week 1: Building Your Sleep Mindset

1. Vandekerckhove, M., Wang, Y.L., 'Emotion, emotion regulation and sleep: An intimate relationship.' *AIMS Neuroscience* 5, 1 (2017): 1–17. doi: 10.3934/Neuroscience.2018.1.1

2. Scott, S. 'Better Believe It.' *Stanford Magazine* (December 2022). stanfordmag.org/contents/better-believe-it

3. Crum, A. J., Salovey, P., Achor, S., 'Rethinking stress: The role of mindsets in determining the stress response.' *Journal of Personality and Social Psychology* 104, 4 (2013): 716–33.

4. Butz, S., Stahlberg, D., 'Can self-compassion improve sleep quality via reduced rumination?' *Self and Identity* 17, 6 (2018): 666–86. doi.org/10.1080/15298868.2018.1456482

5. Li, J., Vitiello, M.V., Gooneratne, N.S., 'Sleep in Normal Aging.' *Sleep Medicine Clinics* 13, 1 (2018): 1–11. doi: 10.1016/j.jsmc.2017.09.001

Mander, B.A., Winer, J.R., Walker, M.P., 'Sleep and Human Aging.' *Neuron* 94, 1 (2017): 19–36. doi: 10.1016/j.neuron.2017.02.004

6. Krause, A.J., Simon, E.B., Mander, B.A., Greer, S.M., Saletin, J.M., Goldstein-Piekarski, A.N., Walker, M.P., 'The sleep-deprived human brain.' *Nature Reviews Neuroscience* 18, 7 (2017): 404–18. doi: 10.1038/nrn.2017.55

7. Lee, M.H., Lee, K.H., Oh, S.M., et al., 'The moderating effect of prefrontal response to sleep-related stimuli on the association between depression and sleep disturbance in insomnia disorder.' *Scientific Reports* 12 (2022), 17739. https://doi.org/10.1038/s41598-022-22652-9

   Regen, W., Kyle, S.D., Nissen, C., Feige, B., Baglioni, C., Hennig, J., Riemann, D., Spiegelhalder, K., 'Objective sleep disturbances are associated with greater waking resting-state connectivity between the retrosplenial cortex/ hippocampus and various nodes of the default mode network.' *Journal of Psychiatry and Neuroscience* 41, 5 (2016): 295–303. doi: 10.1503/jpn.140290

8. Goldberg, S.B., Tucker, R.P., Greene, P.A., Davidson, R.J., Kearney, D.J., Simpson, T.L., 'Mindfulness-based cognitive therapy for the treatment of current depressive symptoms: a meta-analysis.' *Cognitive Behaviour Therapy* 48, 6 (2019): 445–62. doi: 10.1080/16506073.2018.1556330

   Rahrig, H., Vago, D.R., Passarelli, M.A., et al., 'Meta-analytic evidence that mindfulness training alters resting state default mode network connectivity.' *Scientific Reports* 12 (2022). https://doi.org/10.1038/s41598-022-15195-6

9. Transcript of talk by Dr Alia Crum, associate professor of psychology at Stanford University and director of the Stanford Mind & Body Lab, World Economic Forum, 21 February 2018. Quoted in Robson, D. 'How a positive mind really can create a healthier body.' *New Scientist* (27 August 2018), newscientist.com/article/mg23931920-600-mind-over-matter-you-really-can-think-yourself- healthier-and-happier/

10. Gordon, E.M., Chauvin, R.J., Van, A.N., et al., 'A somato-cognitive action network alternates with effector regions in motor cortex.' *Nature* 617 (2023): 351–9. https://doi.org/10.1038/s41586-023-05964-2

11. Béchard, D.E., 'The Huberman Effect.' *Stanford Magazine* (July 2023), https:// stanfordmag.org/contents/the-huberman-effect

   'The Tim Ferriss Show Transcripts: Dr Andrew Huberman – A Neurobiologist on Optimizing Sleep, Performance, and Testosterone (#521).' *Tim Ferriss* (8 July 2021), https://tim.blog/2021/07/08/andrew-huberman-transcript/

12. 'Let Go of Self-Criticism and Discover Self-Compassion.' *Kristin Neff*, self-compassion.org/let-go-of-self-criticism-and-discover-self-compassion/

   Brown, L., Houston, E.E., Amonoo, H.L., et al., 'Is Self-compassion Associated with Sleep Quality? A Meta- analysis.' *Mindfulness* 12 (2021): 82–91. https://doi.org/10.1007/s12671-020-01498-0

   Kirschner, H., Kuyken, W., Wright, K., Roberts, H., Brejcha, C., Karl, A., 'Soothing Your Heart and Feeling Connected: A New Experimental Paradigm to Study the Benefits of Self-Compassion.' *Clinical Psychological Science* 7, 3 (2019): 545–65. https://doi.org/10.1177/2167702618812438

13. Shahar, G., *Erosion: The Psychopathology of Self-Criticism* (Oxford University Press, 2015)

Shahar, G., 'Criticism in the self, brain, social relations and social structure: Implications to psychodynamic psychiatry.' *Psychodynamic Psychiatry* 44, 3 (2016): 395–421. doi: 10.1521/pdps.2016.44.3.395

Shahar, G., 'The Hazards of Self-Criticism: Psychological science sheds light on the detriments of self-derogation.' *Psychology Today* (9 August 2017). https://www.psychologytoday.com/gb/blog/stress-self-and-health/201708/the-hazards-self-criticism

Week 2: Harnessing Circadian Science

1. Borbély, A.A, Daan, S., Wirz-Justice, A., Deboer, T., 'The two-process model of sleep regulation: a reappraisal.' *Journal of Sleep Research* 25, 2 (2016): 131–43. doi: 10.1111/jsr.12371

2. Gillette, M.U., Tischkau, S.A., 'Suprachiasmatic nucleus: the brain's circadian clock.' *Recent Progress in Hormone Research* 54 (1999): 33–58.

3. Ramkisoensing, A., Meijer, J.H., 'Synchronization of biological clock neurons by light and peripheral feedback systems promotes circadian rhythms and health.' *Frontiers in Neurology* 6 (2015): 128. doi: 10.3389/fneur.2015.00128

4. Hayter, E.A., Wehrens, S.M.T., Van Dongen, H.P.A., et al., 'Distinct circadian mechanisms govern cardiac rhythms and susceptibility to arrhythmia.' *Nature Communications* 12, 2472 (2021). https://doi.org/10.1038/s41467- 021-22788-8

5. Zhou, L., Kang, L., Xiao, X., Jia, L., Zhang, Q., Deng, M., '"Gut Microbiota-Circadian Clock Axis" in Deciphering the Mechanism Linking Early-Life Nutritional Environment and Abnormal Glucose Metabolism.' *International Journal of Endocrinology* (2019). doi: 10.1155/2019/5893028

6. Mistlberger, R.E., 'Circadian regulation of sleep in mammals: role of the suprachiasmatic nucleus.' *Brain Research Reviews* 49, 3 (2005): 429–54. doi: 10.1016/j.brainresrev.2005.01.005

7. Duffy, J.F., Cain, S.W., Chang, A.M., Phillips, A.J., Münch, M.Y., Gronfier, C., Wyatt, J.K., Dijk, D.J., Wright, K.P. Jr, Czeisler, C.A., 'Sex difference in the near-24-hour intrinsic period of the human circadian timing system.' *Proceedings of the National Academy of Sciences of the United States of America* 108, Suppl 3 (2011). doi: 10.1073/pnas.1010666108

8. Sahin, L., Wood, B.M., Plitnick, B., Figueiro, M.G., 'Daytime light exposure: Effects on biomarkers, measures of alertness, and performance.' *Behavioural Brain Research* 274 (2014): 176–185.

9. Blume, C., Garbazza, C., Spitschan, M., 'Effects of light on human circadian rhythms, sleep and mood.' *Somnologie (Berl)* 23, 3 (2019): 147–156. doi: 10.1007/s11818-019-00215-x

Waterhouse, J., Fukuda, Y., Morita, T., 'Daily rhythms of the sleep-wake cycle.' *Journal of Physiological Anthropology* 31, 1 (2012). doi: 10.1186/1880-6805-31-5

10. Sullivan Bisson, A.N., Robinson, S.A., Lachman, M.E., 'Walk to a better night of sleep: testing the relationship between physical activity and sleep.' *Sleep Health* 5, 5 (2019): 487–94. doi: 10.1016/j.sleh.2019.06.003

Brown, T.M., 'Melanopic illuminance defines the magnitude of human circadian light responses under a wide range of conditions.' *Journal of Pineal Research* 69, 1 (2020). https://doi.org/10.1111/jpi.12655

11. 'Dr Samer Hattar: Timing Your Light, Food, and Exercise for Optimal Sleep, Energy and Mood. Huberman Lab podcast #43.' *Podcast Disclosed* (22 December 2022). https://podcastdisclosed.com/dr-samer-hattar-timing-your-light-food-exercise-for-optimal-sleep-energy-mood-huberman-lab-podcast-43/

LeGates, T., Fernandez, D., Hattar, S., 'Light as a central modulator of circadian rhythms, sleep and affect.' *Nature Reviews Neuroscience* 15 (2014): 443–54. https://doi.org/10.1038/nrn3743

Shechter, A., Quispe, K.A., Mizhquiri Barbecho, J.S., Slater, C., Falzon, L., 'Interventions to reduce short-wavelength ("blue") light exposure at night and their effects on sleep: A systematic review and meta-analysis.' *SLEEP Advances* 1, 1 (2020). https://doi.org/10.1093/sleepadvances/zpaa002

12. Zhang, Z., Beier, C., Weil, T., et al., 'The retinal ipRGC-preoptic circuit mediates the acute effect of light on sleep.' *Nature Communications* 12 (2021). https://doi.org/10.1038/s41467-021-25378-w

13. Elder, G.J., et al., 'The cortisol awakening response – applications and implications for sleep medicine.' *Sleep Medicine Reviews* 18, 3 (2014): 215–24. doi:10.1016/j.smrv.2013.05.001

Trotti, L.M., 'Waking up is the hardest thing I do all day: Sleep inertia and sleep drunkenness.' *Sleep Medicine Reviews* 35 (2017): 76–84. doi: 10.1016/j.smrv.2016.08.005

14. Blume, C., Garbazza, C., Spitschan, M., 'Effects of light on human circadian rhythms, sleep and mood.' *Somnologie (Berl)* 23, 3 (2019): 147–56. doi: 10.1007/s11818-019-00215-x

Hattar, S., Liao, H.W., Takao, M., Berson, D.M., Yau, K.W., 'Melanopsin-containing retinal ganglion cells: architecture, projections, and intrinsic photosensitivity.' *Science* 295 (2002): 1065–70.

Zhang, Z., Beier, C., Weil, T., Hattar, S., 'The retinal ipRGC-preoptic circuit mediates the acute effect of light on sleep.' *Nature Communications* 12 (2021). https://doi.org/10.1038/s41467-021-25378-w

15. 'Global survey finds we're lacking fresh air and natural light, as we spend less time in nature.' *VELUX* (2019), https://press.velux.com/

new-global-survey-finds-were-lacking-fresh-air-and-natural-light-as-we-spend-less-time-in-nature/

16. Figueiro, M.G., Steverson, B., Heerwagen, J., Kampschroer, K., Hunter, C.M., Gonzales, K., Plitnick, B., Rea, M.S., 'The impact of daytime light exposures on sleep and mood in office workers.' *Sleep Health*. 3, 3 (2017): 204–15. doi: 10.1016/j.sleh.2017.03.005

Schweizer, C., Edwards, R., Bayer-Oglesby, L., et al., 'Indoor time–microenvironment–activity patterns in seven regions of Europe.' *Journal of Exposure Science & Environmental Epidemiology* 17 (2007): 170–81. https://doi.org/10.1038/sj.jes.7500490

Diffey, B.L., 'An overview analysis of the time people spend outdoors.' *British Journal of Dermatology* 164, 4 (2011): 848–54. doi: 10.1111/j.1365-2133.2010.10165.x

17. Choi, K., Shin, C., Kim, T., et al., 'Awakening effects of blue-enriched morning light exposure on university students' physiological and subjective responses.' *Scientific Reports* 9, 345 (2019).

18. Milosavljevic N., 'How Does Light Regulate Mood and Behavioral State?' *Clocks & Sleep* 1, 3 (2019): 319–31. https://doi.org/10.3390/clockssleep1030027

Fernandez, D.C., et al., 'Light Affects Mood and Learning through Distinct Retina-Brain Pathways.' *Cell* 175, 1 (2018). https://doi.org/10.1016/j.cell.2018.08.004

19. Goldstein, A.N., Walker, M.P., 'The Role of Sleep in Emotional Brain Function', *Annual Review of Clinical Psychology* 10, 1 (2014): 679–708.

LeGates, T., Altimus, C., Wang, H., et al., 'Aberrant light directly impairs mood and learning through melanopsin-expressing neurons.' *Nature* 491 (2012), 594–8. https://doi.org/10.1038/nature11673

20. LeGates, T., Fernandez, D., Hattar, S., 'Light as a central modulator of circadian rhythms, sleep and affect.' *Nature Reviews Neuroscience* 15, 443–54 (2014). https://doi.org/10.1038/nrn3743

Blume, C., Garbazza, C., Spitschan, M., 'Effects of light on human circadian rhythms, sleep and mood.' *Somnologie (Berl)* 23, 3 (2019): 147–56. doi: 10.1007/s11818-019-00215-x

Dunster, G.P., et al., 'Daytime light exposure is a strong predictor of seasonal variation in sleep and circadian timing of university students.' *Journal of Pineal Research* (2020). https://doi.org/10.1111/jpi.12843

Estevan, I., Coirolo, N., Tassino, B., Silva, A., 'The Influence of Light and Physical Activity on the Timing and Duration of Sleep: Insights from a Natural Model of Dance Training in Shifts.' *Clocks & Sleep* 5, 1 (2023): 47–61. https://doi.org/10.3390/clockssleep5010006

21. van Egmond, L.T., Titova, O.E., Lindberg, E., et al., 'Association between pet ownership and sleep in the Swedish CArdioPulmonary bioImage Study (*SCAPIS*).' *Scientific Reports* 11 (2021). https://doi.org/10.1038/s41598-021-87080-7

22. Gabel, V., et al., 'Effects of artificial dawn and morning blue light on daytime cognitive performance, well-being, cortisol and melatonin levels.' *Chronobiology International* 30 (2013): 988–97.

    Rahman, S.A., et al., 'Diurnal spectral sensitivity of the acute alerting effects of light.' *Sleep* 37 (2014): 271–81.

    Mead, M.N., 'Benefits of sunlight: a bright spot for human health.' *Environmental Health Perspectives* 116, 4 (2008): A160–7. https://doi.org/10.1289/ehp.116-a160

    Duffy, J.F., Czeisler, C.A., 'Effect of Light on Human Circadian Physiology.' *Sleep Medicine Clinics* 4, 2 (2009): 165–77. doi: 10.1016/j.jsmc.2009.01.004

23. Rosenwasser, A.M., Turek, F.W., 'Neurobiology of Circadian Rhythm Regulation.' *Sleep Medicine Clinics* 10, 4 (2015): 403–12. doi: 10.1016/j.jsmc.2015.08.003

    Golombek, D.A., Rosenstein, R.E., 'Physiology of circadian entrainment.' *Physiological Reviews* 90, 3 (2010): 1063–1102. doi:10.1152/physrev.00009.2009

    Kryger, M.H., Roth, T., Dement, W.C., *Principles and Practice of Sleep Medicine*, 6th edition (Elsevier, 2017)

    'Press Release: 2017 Nobel Prize in Physiology or Medicine awarded jointly to Jeffrey C. Hall, Michael Rosbash and Michael W. Young for their discoveries of molecular mechanisms controlling the circadian rhythm.' *NobelPrize.org* (2 October 2017). https://www.nobelprize.org/prizes/medicine/2017/press-release

24. Melrose, S., 'Seasonal Affective Disorder: An Overview of Assessment and Treatment Approaches.' *Depression Research and Treatment* (2015). doi: 10.1155/2015/178564

25. Lyall, L.M., Wyse, C.A., Celis-Morales, C.A., Lyall, D.M., Cullen, B., Mackay, D., Ward, J., Graham, N., Strawbridge, R.J., Gill, J.M.R., Ferguson, A., Bailey, M.E.S., Pell, J.P., Curtis, A.M., Smith, D.J., 'Seasonality of depressive symptoms in women but not in men: A cross-sectional study in the *UK* Biobank cohort.' *Journal of Affective Disorders* 229 (2018). https://doi.org/10.1016/j.jad.2017.12.106.

26. Nussbaumer-Streit, B., Forneris, C.A., Morgan, L.C., Van Noord, M.G., Gaynes, B.N., Greenblatt, A., Wipplinger, J., Lux, L.J., Winkler, D., Gartlehner, G., 'Light therapy for preventing seasonal affective disorder.' *The Cochrane*

Database of Systematic Reviews 3, 3 (2019). https://pubmed.ncbi.nlm.nih. gov/30883670/

Levitan, R.D., 'What is the optimal implementation of bright light therapy for seasonal affective disorder (SAD)?' *Journal of Psychiatry and Neuroscience* 30, 1 (2005): 72. https://www.ncbi.nlm.nih.gov/pmc/articles/PMC543845/

Virk, G., Reeves, G., Rosenthal, N.E., Sher, L., Postolache, T.T., 'Short exposure to light treatment improves depression scores in patients with seasonal affective disorder: A brief report.' *International Journal on Disability and Human Development* 8, 3 (2009): 283–6. https://pubmed.ncbi.nlm.nih.gov/ 20686638/

27. Chang, A.-M., Aeschbach, D., Duffy, J.F., Czeisler, C.A., 'Evening use of light emitting eReaders negatively affects sleep, circadian timing, and next-morning alertness.' *Proceedings of the National Academy of Sciences of the United States of America* 112 (2015): 1232–7. doi:10.1073/pnas.1418490112

Hysing, M., Pallesen, S., Stormark, K.M., Jakobsen, R., Lundervold, A.J., Sivertsen, B., et al., 'Sleep and use of electronic devices in adolescence: Results from a large population-based study.' *BMJ Open* 5 (2015). doi:10.1136/ bmjopen-2014-006748

Fonken, L.K., Workman, J.L., Walton, J.C., Weil, Z.M., Morris, J.S., Haim, A., Nelson, R.J., 'Light at night increases body mass by shifting the time of food intake.' *Proceedings of the National Academy of Sciences of the United States of America* 107, 43 (2010): 18664–9. https://pubmed.ncbi.nlm.nih. gov/20937863/

Sancar, A., Lindsey-Boltz, L.A., Gaddameedhi, S., Selby, C.P., Ye, R., Chiou, Y.Y., Kemp, M.G., Hu, J., Lee, J.H., Ozturk, N., 'Circadian clock, cancer, and chemotherapy.' *Biochemistry* 54, 2 (2015): 110–23. https://pubmed. ncbi.nlm.nih.gov/25302769/

Wahl, S., Engelhardt, M., Schaupp, P., Lappe, C., Ivanov, I.V., 'The inner clock: Blue light sets the human rhythm.' *Journal of Biophotonics* 12, 12 (2019). https://pubmed.ncbi.nlm.nih.gov/31433569/

Vandewalle, G., Maquet, P., Dijk, D.J., 'Light as a modulator of cognitive brain function.' *Trends in Cognitive Sciences* 13, 10 (2009): 429–38. https:// linkinghub.elsevier.com/retrieve/pii/S1364661309001685

28. Tordjman, S., Chokron, S., Delorme, R., Charrier. A., Bellissant, E., Jaafari, N., et al., 'Melatonin: Pharmacology, functions and therapeutic benefits.' *Current Neuropharmacology* 15 (2017): 434–43. 10.2174/1570159X14666161228122115

Lockley, S.W., Brainard, G.C., Czeisler, C.A., 'High sensitivity of the human circadian melatonin rhythm to resetting by short wavelength light.' *The Journal of Clinical Endocrinology and Metabolism* 88, 9 (2003): 4502–5. https:// academic.oup.com/jcem/article/88/9/4502/2845835

29. 'Blue light has a dark side.' *Harvard Health Publishing* (7 July 2020).
      https://www.health.harvard.edu/staying-healthy/blue-light-has-a-dark-side
      Kayumov, L., Casper, R.F., Hawa, R.J., Perelman, B., Chung, S.A.,
      Sokalsky, S., Shapiro, C.M., 'Blocking Low-Wavelength Light Prevents Noc-
      turnal Melatonin Suppression with No Adverse Effect on Performance during
      Simulated Shift Work.' *The Journal of Clinical Endocrinology and Metabolism* 90,
      5 (2005): 2755–61. https://doi.org/10.1210/jc.2004-2062

30. Erickson, M., 'Setting your biological clock, reducing stress while sheltering in
      place.' *Scope (Stanford Medicine)* (3 June 2020). https://scopeblog.stanford.
      edu/2020/06/03/setting-your-biological-clock-reducing-stress-while-
      sheltering-in-place/#:~:text=The%20eye%20and%20brain%20clocks,have%
      20flown%20to%20Abu%20Dhabi.%22

31. Molen, Y., Santos, G., Carvalho, L., Prado, L., Prado, G., 'Pre-sleep worry
      decrease by adding reading and guided imagery to insomnia treatment.' *Sleep
      Medicine* 14, 1 (2013): e210–e211. https://doi.org/10.1016/j.sleep.2013.11.504
      'Reading is good for you.' *Royal Holloway Weekly Wellbeing Focus,*
      https://intranet.royalholloway.ac.uk/staff/your-employment/human-
      resources/organisation-development/working-well-from-home/
      weekly-wellbeing-focus-reading-is-good-for-you.aspx
      'Reading "can help reduce stress"' *Telegraph* (30 March 2009). https://
      www.telegraph.co.uk/news/health/news/5070874/Reading-can-help-reduce-
      stress.html
      Finucane, E., O'Brien, A., Treweek, S., et al., 'Does reading a book in bed
      make a difference to sleep in comparison to not reading a book in bed? The
      People's Trial—an online, pragmatic, randomised trial.' *Trials* 22, 873 (2021).
      https://doi.org/10.1186/s13063-021-05831-3

32. Dolan, E.W., 'Preliminary Study of the Psychophysiological Effects of Texting.'
      PsyPost (25 May 2010). https://www.psypost.org/2010/05/psychophysiological-
      effect-texting-842
      Oksenberg, A., Silverberg, D.S., 'The effect of body posture on sleep-
      related breathing disorders: facts and therapeutic implications.' *Sleep Medicine
      Reviews* 2, 3 (1998): 139–62. https://doi.org/10.1016/S1087-0792(98)
      90018-1

33. Chervin, R.D., Ruzicka, D.L., Giordani, B.J., Weatherly, R.A., Dillon, J.E.,
      Hodges, E.K., et al., 'Sleep- disordered breathing, behavior, and cognition in
      children before and after adenotonsillectomy.' *Pediatrics* 117 (2006): e769–
      e778. doi: 10.1542/peds.2005-1837

34. Woods, H.C., Scott, H., '#Sleepyteens: Social media use in adolescence is asso-
      ciated with poor sleep quality, anxiety, depression and low self-esteem.' *Journal
      of Adolescence* 51 (2016): 41–9. doi: 10.1016/j.adolescence.2016.05.008

Cain, N., Gradisar, M., 'Electronic media use and sleep in school-aged children and adolescents: a review.' *Sleep Medicine* 11 (2010): 735–42. doi:10.1016/j.sleep.2010.02.006

Lund, L., Sølvhøj, I.N., Danielsen, D., et al., 'Electronic media use and sleep in children and adolescents in Western countries: a systematic review.' *BMC Public Health* 21, 1598 (2021). https://doi.org/10.1186/s12889-021-11640-9

Calamaro, C.J., Mason, T.B., Ratcliffe, S.J., 'Adolescents living the 24/7 lifestyle: effects of caffeine and technology on sleep duration and daytime functioning.' *Pediatrics* 123 (2009): e1005–10. doi: 10.1542/peds.2008-3641

35. van der Lely, S., Frey, S., Garbazza, C., Wirz-Justice, A., Jenni, O.G., Steiner, R., et al., 'Blue blocker glasses as a countermeasure for alerting effects of evening light-emitting diode screen exposure in male teenagers.' *Journal of Adolescent Health* 56 (2015): 113–19.

Sasseville, A., Paquet, N., Sevigny, J., Hebert, M., 'Blue blocker glasses impede the capacity of bright light to suppress melatonin production.' *Journal of Pineal Research* 41 (2006): 73–8.

36. Hysing, M., Pallesen, S., Stormark, K.M., et al, 'Sleep and use of electronic devices in adolescence: results from a large population-based study.' *BMJ Open* 5 (2015). doi: 10.1136/bmjopen-2014-006748

Gradisar, M., Gardner, G., Dohnt, H., 'Recent worldwide sleep patterns and problems during adolescence: a review and meta-analysis of age, region, and sleep.' *Sleep Medicine* 12 (2011): 110–18. doi: 10.1016/j.sleep.2010.11.008

37. Maruani, J.P., Geoffroy, A., 'Bright Light as a Personalized Precision Treatment of Mood Disorders.' *Frontiers in Psychiatry* 10 (2019). https://doi.org/10.3389/fpsyt.2019.00085

38. Brinkman, J.E., Reddy, V., Sharma, S., 'Physiology of Sleep.' *StatPearls* (2023). https://www.ncbi.nlm.nih.gov/books/NBK482512/

Saper, C.B., Chou, T.C., Scammell, T.E., 'The sleep switch: hypothalamic control of sleep and wakefulness.' *Trends in Neurosciences* 24, 12 (2001): 726–31.

Memar, P., Faradji, F.A., 'Novel Multi-Class *EEG*-Based Sleep Stage Classification System.' *IEEE Transactions on Neural Systems and Rehabilitation Engineering* 26, 1 (2018): 84–95.

Patel, A.K., Reddy, V., Shumway, K.R., et al., 'Physiology, Sleep Stages.' *StatPearls* (2023). https://www.ncbi.nlm.nih.gov/books/NBK526132/

39. 'Brain basics: Understanding sleep.' *National Institute of Neurological Disorders and Stroke* (2022). https://www.ninds.nih.gov/health-information/patient-caregiver-education/brain-basics-understanding-sleep

Schönauer, M., Pöhlchen, D., 'Sleep spindles.' *Current Biology* 28, 19 (2018): R1129–R1130. https://pubmed.ncbi.nlm.nih.gov/30300592/

40. Walker, M.P., 'The role of sleep in cognition and emotion.' *Annals of the New York Academy of Sciences* 1156 (2009):168–97.

Mantua, J., 'Sleep Physiology Correlations and Human Memory Consolidation: Where Do We Go From Here?' *Sleep* 41, 2 (2018). https://doi.org/10.1093/sleep/zsx204

Walker, M.P., van der Helm, E., 'Overnight therapy? The role of sleep in emotional brain processing.' *Psychological Bulletin* 135, 5 (2009): 731–48. doi: 10.1037/a0016570

41. Tamaki, M., Wang, Z., Barnes-Diana, T., et al., 'Complementary contributions of non-REM and REM sleep to visual learning.' *Nature Neuroscience* 23 (2020): 1150–6. https://doi.org/10.1038/s41593-020-0666-y

42. Skurvydas, A., Zlibinaite, L., Solianik, R., Brazaitis, M., Valanciene, D., Baranauskiene, N., Majauskiene, D., Mickeviciene, D., Venckunas, T., Kamandulis, S., 'One night of sleep deprivation impairs executive function but does not affect psychomotor or motor performance.' *Biology of Sport* 37, 1 (2020): 7–14. doi: 10.5114/biolsport.2020.89936

43. Vartanian, O., Bouak, F., Caldwell, J.L., Cheung, B., Cupchik, G., Jobidon, M-E., Lam, Q., Nakashima, A., Paul, M., Peng, H., Silvia, P.J., Smith, I., 'The effects of a single night of sleep deprivation on fluency and prefrontal cortex function during divergent thinking.' *Frontiers in Human Neuroscience* 8 (2014): 214. doi: 10.3389/fnhum.2014.00214

Nir, Y., Andrillon, T., Marmelshtein, A., et al., 'Selective neuronal lapses precede human cognitive lapses following sleep deprivation.' *Nature Medicine* 23 (2017): 1474–80. https://doi.org/10.1038/nm.4433

44. Mander, B.A., et al., 'Wake Deterioration and Sleep Restoration of Human Learning.' *Current Biology* 21, 5 (2011). doi:10.1016/j.cub.2011.01.019

Walker, M.P., 'The role of slow wave sleep in memory processing.' *Journal of Clinical Sleep Medicine*, 5, Suppl 2 (2009): S20–S26.

Walker, M.P., et al., 'Cognitive Flexibility across the Sleep–Wake Cycle: REM-Sleep Enhancement of Anagram Problem Solving.' *Cognitive Brain Research* 14, 3 (2002): 317–24. doi:10.1016/s0926-6410(02)00134-9

Chiang, Y.C., Arendt, S.W., 'Benefits of Sleep for Undergraduate Students' Academic Performance.' *Journal of Hospitality Tourism Education* 29, 2 (2017): 61–70. doi: 10.1080/10963758.2017.1297713

45. Colten, H.R., Altevogt, B.M., editors., 'Sleep Physiology'. In *Sleep Disorders and Sleep Deprivation: An Unmet Public Health Problem*. (Institute of Medicine (US) Committee on Sleep Medicine and Research, National Academies Press, 2006). doi: 10.17226/11617

46. Islam, Z., Hu, H., Akter, S., Kuwahara, K., Kochi, T., Eguchi, M., Kurotani, K., Nanri, A., Kabe, I., Mizoue, T., 'Social jetlag is associated with an increased likelihood of having depressive symptoms among the Japanese working population: the Furukawa Nutrition and Health Study.' *Sleep* 43, 1 (2020). https://doi.org/10.1093/sleep/zsz204

Wittmann, M., Dinich, J., Merrow, M., Roenneberg, T., 'Social jetlag: misalignment of biological and social time.' *Chronobiology International* 23, 1–2 (2006): 497–509. doi: 10.1080/07420520500545979

Acosta, J., Crespo, M.T., Plano, S.A., Golombek, D.A., Chiesa, J.J., Agostino, P.V., 'Chronic jet lag reduces motivation and affects other mood-related behaviors in male mice.' *Frontiers in Physiology* 14 (2023). doi: 10.3389/fphys.2023.1225134

Caliandro, R., Streng, A.A., van Kerkhof, L.W.M., van der Horst, G.T.J., Chaves, I., 'Social Jetlag and Related Risks for Human Health: A Timely Review.' *Nutrients* 13, 12 (2021): 4543. https://doi.org/10.3390/nu13124543

American Academy of Sleep Medicine, 'Social jet lag is associated with worse mood, poorer health and heart disease.' *ScienceDaily* (5 June 2017). https://www.sciencedaily.com/releases/2017/06/170605085326.htm

47. Bermingham, K.M., Stensrud, S., Asnicar, F., et al., 'Exploring the relationship between social jetlag with gut microbial composition, diet and cardiometabolic health, in the *ZOE PREDICT* 1 cohort.' *European Journal of Nutrition* (2023). https://doi.org/10.1007/s00394-023-03204-x

O'Loughlin, J., Casanova, F., Jones, S.E., et al., 'Using Mendelian Randomisation methods to understand whether diurnal preference is causally related to mental health.' *Molecular Psychiatry* 26 (2021): 6305–16. https://doi.org/10.1038/s41380-021-01157-3

48. Hena, M., Garmy, P., 'Social Jetlag and Its Association With Screen Time and Nighttime Texting Among Adolescents in Sweden: A Cross-Sectional Study.' *Frontiers in Neuroscience* 14 (2020): 122. doi: 10.3389/fnins.2020.00122

O'Loughlin, J., Casanova, F., Jones, S.E., et al., 'Using Mendelian Randomisation methods to understand whether diurnal preference is causally related to mental health.' *Molecular Psychiatry* 26 (2021): 6305–16. https://doi.org/10.1038/s41380-021-01157-3

Korman, M., Tkachev, V., Reis, C., et al., 'COVID-19-mandated social restrictions unveil the impact of social time pressure on sleep and body clock.' *Scientific Reports* 10 (2020). https://doi.org/10.1038/s41598-020-79299-7

'"Social Jetlag" Measured by Differences in Sleep Patterns on Days Off Vs. Work Days, Associated with Poor Overall Health.' *The University of Arizona College of Medicine* (5 June 2017). https://medicine.arizona.edu/news/2017/

ua-research-social-jetlag-measured-differences-sleep-patterns-days-vs-work-days-associated

49. Kalmbach, D., Schneider, L.D., Cheung, J., Bertrand, S.J., Kariharan, T., Pack, A.I, Gehrman, P.R., 'Genetic Basis of Chronotype in Humans: Insights From Three Landmark GWAS.' *Sleep* 40, 2 (2017). https://doi.org/10.1093/sleep/zsw048

    Jones, S.E., Lane, J.M., Wood, A.R., van Hees V.T., Tyrrell, J., Beaumont, R.N., et al, 'Genome-wide association analyses of chronotype in 697,828 individuals provides insights into circadian rhythms.' *Nature Communications* 10 (2019): 343.

50. Cordi, M.J., Schlarb, A.A., Rasch, B., 'Deepening sleep by hypnotic suggestion.' *Sleep* 37, 6 (2014): 1143–52. doi: 10.5665/sleep.3778

    Cordi, M.J., Ackermann, S., Rasch, B., 'Effects of Relaxing Music on Healthy Sleep.' *Scientific Reports* 9, 1 (2019): 9079. doi: 10.1038/s41598-019-45608-y

    Cordi, M.J., Rossier, L., Rasch, B., 'Hypnotic suggestions given before nighttime sleep extend slow-wave sleep as compared to a control text in highly hypnotizable subjects.' *International Journal of Clinical and Experimental Hypnosis* 68, 1 (2020): 105–29. doi: 10.1080/00207144.2020.1687260

Week 3: Fuelling Your Sleep Well-Being

1. St-Onge, M-P., O'Keeffe, M., Roberts, A.L., RoyChoudhury, A., Laferrère, B., 'Short Sleep Duration, Glucose Dysregulation and Hormonal Regulation of Appetite in Men and Women.' *Sleep* 35, 11 (2012). https://doi.org/10.5665/sleep.2198

    Tsereteli, N., Vallat, R., Fernandez-Tajes, J., et al., 'Impact of insufficient sleep on dysregulated blood glucose control under standardised meal conditions.' *Diabetologia* 65 (2022): 356–65. https://doi.org/10.1007/s00125-021-05608-y

    Ndahimana, D., Kim, E.K., 'Measurement Methods for Physical Activity and Energy Expenditure: a Review.' *Clinical Nutrition Research* 6, 2 (2017): 68–80. https://doi.org/10.7762/cnr.2017.6.2.68

    Greer, S., Goldstein, A., Walker, M., 'The impact of sleep deprivation on food desire in the human brain.' *Nature Communications* 4 (2013). https://doi.org/10.1038/ncomms3259

2. Hall, H., Perelman, D., Breschi, A., Limcaoco, P., Kellogg, R., McLaughlin, T., et al., 'Glucotypes reveal new patterns of glucose dysregulation.' *PLoS Biology* 16, 7 (2018). https://doi.org/10.1371/journal.pbio.2005143

3. Taheri, S., Lin, L., Austin, D., Young, T., Mignot, E., 'Short sleep duration is associated with reduced leptin, elevated ghrelin, and increased body mass index.' *PLoS Medicine* 1, 3 (2004). doi: 10.1371/journal.pmed.0010062

4. Taheri, S., Lin, L., Austin, D., Young, T., Mignot, E., 'Short sleep duration is associated with reduced leptin, elevated ghrelin, and increased body mass index.' *PLoS Medicine* 1, 3 (2004). doi: 10.1371/journal.pmed.0010062

   St-Onge, M.P., 'Sleep-obesity relation: underlying mechanisms and consequences for treatment.' *Obesity Reviews* 18, Suppl 1 (2017): 34–9. doi: 10.1111/obr.12499

5. Al Khatib, H.K., Harding, S.V., Darzi, J., Pot, G.K., 'The effects of partial sleep deprivation on energy balance: a systematic review and meta-analysis.' *European Journal of Clinical Nutrition* 71, 5 (2017): 614–24. doi: 10.1038/ejcn.2016.201

6. Benjamins, J.S., Hooge, I.T.C., Benedict, C., Smeets, P.A.M., van der Laan, L.N., 'The influence of acute partial sleep deprivation on liking, choosing and consuming high- and low-energy foods.' *Food Quality and Preference* 88 (2021). https://doi.org/10.1016/j.foodqual.2020.104074.

   Grandner, M.A., Seixas, A., Shetty, S., et al., 'Sleep Duration and Diabetes Risk: Population Trends and Potential Mechanisms.' *Current Diabetes Reports* 16, 106 (2016). https://doi.org/10.1007/s11892-016-0805-8

7. Knutson, K.L., 'Impact of Sleep and Sleep Loss on Glucose Homeostasis and Appetite Regulation.' *Sleep Medicine Clinics* 2, 2 (2007): 187–97. https://doi.org/10.1016/j.jsmc.2007.03.004

   Scheen, A.J., Byrne, M.M., Plat, L., Leproult, R., Van Cauter, E., 'Relationships between sleep quality and glucose regulation in normal humans.' *American Journal of Physiology* 271, 2 Pt 1 (1996): E261–70. doi: 10.1152/ajpendo.1996.271.2.E261

8. Buffey, A.J., Herring, M.P., Langley, C.K., et al., 'The Acute Effects of Interrupting Prolonged Sitting Time in Adults with Standing and Light-Intensity Walking on Biomarkers of Cardiometabolic Health in Adults: A Systematic Review and Meta-analysis.' *Sports Medicine* 52 (2022): 1765–87. https://doi.org/10.1007/s40279-022-01649-4

   Vincent, G.E., Gupta, C.C., Sprajcer, M., Vandelanotte, C., Duncan, M.J., Tucker, P., Lastella, M., Tuckwell, G.A., Ferguson, S.A., 'Are prolonged sitting and sleep restriction a dual curse for the modern workforce? A randomised controlled trial protocol.' *BMJ Open* 10, 7 (2020). doi: 10.1136/bmjopen-2020-040613

9. Sullivan Bisson, A.N., Robinson, S.A., Lachman, M.E., 'Walk to a better night of sleep: testing the relationship between physical activity and sleep.' *Sleep Health* 5, 5 (2019): 487–94. doi: 10.1016/j.sleh.2019.06.003

   Brown, D.K., Barton, J.L., Gladwell, V.F., 'Viewing nature scenes positively affects recovery of autonomic function following acute-mental stress.' *Environmental Science and Technology* 47, 11 (2013): 5562–9. doi: 10.1021/es305019p

10. 'This is Your Brain on Sleep, Supplements, Sunlight, and Stimulation – Stanford Neuroscientist Andrew Huberman, PhD.' *The Kevin Rose Show* (14 February 2021). https://podcast.kevinrose.com/this-is-your-brain-on-sleep-supplements-sunlight-and-stimulation-stanford-neuroscientist-andrew-huberman-phd/

11. Stich, F.M., et al., 'The potential role of sleep in promoting a healthy body composition: underlying mechanisms determining muscle, fat, and bone mass and their association with sleep.' *Neuroendocrinology* 112, 7 (2022): 673–701. https://www.karger.com/Article/FullText/518691

12. Berry, S.E., Valdes, A.M., Drew, D.A., et al., 'Human postprandial responses to food and potential for precision nutrition.' *Nature Medicine* 26 (2020): 964–73. https://doi.org/10.1038/s41591-020-0934-0

    Tsereteli, N., Vallat, R., Fernandez-Tajes, J., et al., 'Impact of insufficient sleep on dysregulated blood glucose control under standardised meal conditions.' *Diabetologia* 65 (2022): 356–65. https://doi.org/10.1007/s00125-021-05608-y

13. Vallat, R., Berry, S.E., Tsereteli, N., et al., 'How people wake up is associated with previous night's sleep together with physical activity and food intake.' *Nature Communications* 13 (2022). https://doi.org/10.1038/s41467-022-34503-2

14. Frank, S., Gonzalez, K., Lee-Ang, L., et al., 'Diet and sleep physiology: public health and clinical implications.' *Frontiers in Neurology* 8 (2017): 393. doi:10.3389/fneur.2017.00393.

    Binks, H., Vincent, G.E., Gupta, C., Irwin, C., Khalesi, S., 'Effects of Diet on Sleep: A Narrative Review.' *Nutrients* 12, 4 (2020): 936. https://doi.org/10.3390/nu12040936

    Chaput, J.P., 'Sleep patterns, diet quality and energy balance.' *Physiology and Behavior* 134 (2014): 86–91. doi:10.1016/j.physbeh.2013.09.006

    Peuhkuri, K., Sihvola, N., Korpela, R., 'Diet promotes sleep duration and quality.' *Nutrition Research* 32 (2012): 309–19. doi: 10.1016/j.nutres.2012.03.009

15. Godos, J., Ferri, R., Castellano, S., Angelino, D., Mena, P., Del Rio, D., Caraci, F., Galvano, F., Grosso, G., 'Specific Dietary (Poly)phenols Are Associated with Sleep Quality in a Cohort of Italian Adults.' *Nutrients* 12, 5 (2020): 1226. https://doi.org/10.3390/nu12051226

    Kanagasabai, T., Ardern, C.I., 'Inflammation, Oxidative Stress, and Antioxidants Contribute to Selected Sleep Quality and Cardiometabolic Health Relationships: A Cross-Sectional Study.' *Mediators of Inflammation* (2015).

    Kanagasabai, T., Ardern, C.I., 'Contribution of Inflammation, Oxidative Stress, and Antioxidants to the Relationship between Sleep Duration and Cardiometabolic Health.' *Sleep* 38 (2015): 1905–12.

St-Onge, M.P., Crawford, A., Aggarwal, B., 'Plant-based diets: Reducing cardiovascular risk by improving sleep quality.' *Current Sleep Medicine Reports* 4, 1 (2018): 74–8.

Wang, X., Song, F., Wang, B., et al., 'Vegetarians have an indirect positive effect on sleep quality through depression condition.' *Scientific Reports* 13 (2023). https://doi.org/10.1038/s41598-023-33912-7

16. Höglund, E., Øverli, Ø., Winberg, S., 'Tryptophan Metabolic Pathways and Brain Serotonergic Activity: A Comparative Review.' *Frontiers in Endocrinology* 10 (2019): 158. doi: 10.3389/fendo.2019.00158

Zhao, D., Yu, Y., Shen, Y., Liu, Q., Zhao, Z., Sharma, R., Reiter, R.J., 'Melatonin Synthesis and Function: Evolutionary History in Animals and Plants.' *Frontiers in Endocrinology* 10 (2019): 249. doi: 10.3389/fendo.2019.00249

Martínez-Rodríguez, A., Rubio-Arias, J.Á., Ramos-Campo, D.J., Reche-García, C., Leyva-Vela, B., Nadal-Nicolás, Y., 'Psychological and Sleep Effects of Tryptophan and Magnesium-Enriched Mediterranean Diet in Women with Fibromyalgia.' *International Journal of Environmental Research and Public Health* 17, 7 (2020): 2227. doi: 10.3390/ijerph17072227

Mantantzis, K., Campos, V., Darimont, C., Martin, F.P., 'Effects of Dietary Carbohydrate Profile on Nocturnal Metabolism, Sleep, and Wellbeing: A Review.' *Frontiers in Public Health* 10 (2022). doi: 10.3389/fpubh.2022.931781

17. Dashti, H.S., Follis, J.L., Smith, C.E., et al., 'Habitual sleep duration is associated with *BMI* and macronutrient intake and may be modified by *CLOCK* genetic variants.' *The American Journal of Clinical Nutrition* 101 (2015): 135–43.

Jahangard, L., Sadeghi, A., Ahmadpanah, M., et al., 'Influence of adjuvant omega-3-polyunsaturated fatty acids on depression, sleep, and emotion regulation among outpatients with major depressive disorders—results from a double-blind, randomized and placebo-controlled clinical trial.' *Journal of Psychiatric Research* 107 (2018): 48–56.

18. Montgomery, P., Burton, J.R., Sewell, R.P., Spreckelsen, T.F., Richardson, A.J., 'Fatty acids and sleep in UK children: subjective and pilot objective sleep results from the DOLAB study – a randomized controlled trial.' *Journal of Sleep Research* 23, 4 (2014): 364–88. https://doi.org/10.1111/jsr.12135

Murphy, R., Devarshi, P.P., Mun, J.G., Marshall, K., Mitmesser, S.H., 'Association of omega-3 levels and sleep in US adults, National Health and Nutrition Examination Survey, 2011–2012.' *Sleep Health* 8, 3 (2022): 294–7. https://doi.org/10.1016/j.sleh.2021.12.003

19. Hansen, A.L., Dahl, L., Olson, G., Thornton, D., Graff, I.E., Frøyland, L., Thayer, J.F., Pallesen, S., 'Fish consumption, sleep, daily functioning, and heart rate variability.' *Journal of Clinical Sleep Medicine* 10, 5 (2014): 567–75. doi: 10.5664/jcsm.3714

Murphy, R., Devarshi, P.P., Mun, J.G., Marshall, K., Mitmesser, S.H., 'Association of omega-3 levels and sleep in US adults, National Health and Nutrition Examination Survey, 2011–2012.' *Sleep Health* 8, 3 (2022): 294–7. https://doi.org/10.1016/j.sleh.2021.12.003

20. Patrick, R.P., Ames, B.N., 'Vitamin D and the omega-3 fatty acids control serotonin synthesis and action, part 2: relevance for ADHD, bipolar disorder, schizophrenia, and impulsive behavior.' *The FASEB Journal* 29, 6 (2015): 2207–22. doi:10.1096/fj.14-268342

21. Montgomery, P., Burton, J.R., Sewell, R.P., Spreckelsen, T.F., Richardson, A.J., 'Fatty acids and sleep in *UK* children: subjective and pilot objective sleep results from the *DOLAB* study – a randomized controlled trial.' *Journal of Sleep Research* 23, 4 (2014): 364–88. https://doi.org/10.1111/jsr.12135

22. Wilson, K., St-Onge, M.P., Tasali, E., 'Diet Composition and Objectively Assessed Sleep Quality: A Narrative Review.' *Journal of the Academy of Nutrition and Dietetics* 122, 6 (2022): 1182–95. doi: 10.1016/j.jand.2022.01.007

   Sutanto, C.N., Loh, W.W., Toh, D.W.K., Lee, D.P.S., Kim, J.E., 'Association Between Dietary Protein Intake and Sleep Quality in Middle-Aged and Older Adults in Singapore.' *Frontiers in Nutrition* 9 (2022). doi: 10.3389/fnut.2022.832341. *PMID*: 35356724; *PMCID*: *PMC8959711*.

23. Tanaka, E., Yatsuya, H., Uemura, M., Murata, C., Otsuka, R., Toyoshima, H., Tamakoshi, K., Sasaki, S., Kawaguchi, L., Aoyama, A., 'Associations of protein, fat, and carbohydrate intakes with insomnia symptoms among middle-aged Japanese workers.' *Journal of Epidemiology* 23, 2 (2013): 132–8. doi: 10.2188/jea.je20120101

   Dragana, R., et al., 'A gut-secreted peptide suppresses arousability from sleep.' *Cell* 186, 7 (2023): 1382–97. doi: 10.1016/j.cell.2023.02.022

   Brandão, L.E.M., Popa, A., Cedernaes, E., Cedernaes, C., Lampola, L., Cedernaes, J., 'Exposure to a more unhealthy diet impacts sleep microstructure during normal sleep and recovery sleep: A randomized trial.' *Obesity* 31, 7 (2023): 1755–66. doi:10.1002/oby.23787

24. Lin, H.H., Tsai, P.S., Fang, S.C., Liu, J.F., 'Effect of kiwifruit consumption on sleep quality in adults with sleep problems.' *Asia Pacific Journal of Clinical Nutrition* 20, 2 (2011): 169–74.

   Thompson, R.S., Vargas, F., Dorrestein, P.C., et al., 'Dietary prebiotics alter novel microbial dependent fecal metabolites that improve sleep.' *Scientific Reports* 10 (2020). https://doi.org/10.1038/s41598-020-60679-y

25. Pigeon, W.R., Carr, M., Gorman, C., Perlis, M.L., 'Effects of a tart cherry juice beverage on the sleep of older adults with insomnia: a pilot study.' *Journal of Medicinal Food* 13, 3 (2010): 579–83. doi: 10.1089/jmf.2009.0096.

   Howatson, G., Bell, P.G., Tallent, J., Middleton, B., McHugh, M.P., Ellis, J., 'Effect of tart cherry juice (Prunus cerasus) on melatonin levels and enhanced sleep quality.' *European Journal of Nutrition* 51, 8 (2012): 909–16. doi: 10.1007/s00394-011-0263-7

26. Losso, J.N., Finley, J.W., Karki, N., Liu, A.G., Prudente, A., Tipton, R., Yu, Y., Greenway, F.L., 'Pilot Study of the Tart Cherry Juice for the Treatment of Insomnia and Investigation of Mechanisms.' *American Journal of Therapeutics* 25, 2 (2018): e194–e201. doi: 10.1097/MJT.0000000000000584

27. Yoto, A., Motoki, M., Murao, S., et al., 'Effects of L-theanine or caffeine intake on changes in blood pressure under physical and psychological stresses.' *Journal of Physiological Anthropology* 31, 28 (2012). https://doi.org/10.1186/1880-6805-31-28

28. Hidese, S., Ogawa, S., Ota, M., Ishida, I., Yasukawa, Z., Ozeki, M., Kunugi, H., 'Effects of L-Theanine Administration on Stress-Related Symptoms and Cognitive Functions in Healthy Adults: A Randomized Controlled Trial.' *Nutrients* 11, 10 (2019): 2362. doi: 10.3390/nu11102362

   Rao, T.P., Ozeki, M., Juneja, L.R., 'In Search of a Safe Natural Sleep Aid.' *Journal of the American College of Nutrition* 34, 5 (2015): 436–47. doi: 10.1080/07315724.2014.926153

29. Qiu, Y., Mao, Z.J., Ruan, Y.P., Zhang, X., 'Exploration of the anti-insomnia mechanism of Ganoderma by central-peripheral multi-level interaction network analysis.' *BMC Microbiology* 21, 1 (2021): 296. doi: 10.1186/s12866-021-02361-5

30. Yao, C., Wang, Z., Jiang, H., et al., 'Ganoderma lucidum promotes sleep through a gut microbiota-dependent and serotonin-involved pathway in mice.' *Scientific Reports* 11 (2021). https://doi.org/10.1038/s41598-021-92913-6

   Chu, Q.P., Wang, L.E., Cui, X.Y., Fu, H.Z., Lin, Z.B., Lin, S.Q., Zhang, Y.H., 'Extract of Ganoderma lucidum potentiates pentobarbital-induced sleep via a GABAergic mechanism.' *Pharmacology Biochemistry and Behavior* 86, 4 (2007): 693–8. doi: 10.1016/j.pbb.2007.02.015

31. Chu, Q.P., Wang, L.E., Cui, X.Y., Fu, H.Z., Lin, Z.B., Lin, S.Q., Zhang, Y.H., 'Extract of Ganoderma lucidum potentiates pentobarbital-induced sleep via a GABAergic mechanism.' *Pharmacology Biochemistry and Behavior* 86, 4 (2007): 693–8. doi: 10.1016/j.pbb.2007.02.015

32. Cui, X.Y., Cui, S.Y., Zhang, J., Wang, Z.J., Yu, B., Sheng, Z.F., Zhang, X.Q., Zhang, Y.H., 'Extract of Ganoderma lucidum prolongs sleep time in rats.' *Journal of Ethnopharmacology* 139, 3 (2012): 796–800. doi: 10.1016/j.jep.2011.12.020

33. Tang, W., Gao, Y., Chen, G., Gao, H., Dai, X., Ye, J., Chan, E., Huang, M., Zhou, S., 'A randomized, double-blind and placebo-controlled study of a Ganoderma lucidum polysaccharide extract in neurasthenia.' *Journal of Medicinal Food* 8, 1 (2005): 53–8. doi: 10.1089/jmf.2005.8.53

34. Held, K., Antonijevic, I.A., Künzel, H., Uhr, M., Wetter, T.C., Golly, I.C., Steiger, A., Murck, H., 'Oral Mg(2+) supplementation reverses age-related neuroendocrine and sleep EEG changes in humans.' *Pharmacopsychiatry* 35, 4 (2002): 135–43. doi: 10.1055/s-2002-33195

    Abbasi, B., Kimiagar, M., Sadeghniiat, K., Shirazi, M.M., Hedayati, M., Rashidkhani, B., 'The effect of magnesium supplementation on primary insomnia in elderly: A double-blind placebo-controlled clinical trial.' *Journal of Research in Medical Sciences* 17, 12 (2012): 1161–9.

    Zhang, Y., Chen, C., Lu, L., Knutson, K.L., Carnethon, M.R., Fly, A.D., Luo, J., Haas, D.M., Shikany, J.M., Kahe, K., 'Association of magnesium intake with sleep duration and sleep quality: findings from the *CARDIA* study.' *Sleep* 45, 4 (2022). doi: 10.1093/sleep/zsab276

    Ju, S.Y., Choi, W.S., Ock, S.M., Kim, C.M., Kim, D.H., 'Dietary magnesium intake and metabolic syndrome in the adult population: dose-response meta-analysis and meta-regression.' *Nutrients* 6, 12 (2014): 6005–19. doi: 10.3390/nu6126005

35. Mah, J., Pitre, T., 'Oral magnesium supplementation for insomnia in older adults: a Systematic Review & Meta-Analysis.' *BMC Complementary Medicine and Therapies* 21, 125 (2021). https://doi.org/10.1186/s12906-021-03297-z

36. Nielsen, F.H., Johnson, L.K., Zeng, H., 'Magnesium supplementation improves indicators of low magnesium status and inflammatory stress in adults older than 51 years with poor quality sleep.' *Magnesium Research* 23, 4 (2010): 158–68. doi: 10.1684/mrh.2010.0220

37. Ghabriel, M.N., Vink, R., 'Magnesium transport across the blood-brain barriers.' In: Vink, R., Nechifor, M., editors, *Magnesium in the Central Nervous System.* (University of Adelaide Press, 2011).

    Zhang, C., Hu, Q., Li, S., Dai, F., Qian, W., Hewlings, S., Yan, T., Wang, Y., 'A Magtein®, Magnesium L-Threonate, -Based Formula Improves Brain Cognitive Functions in Healthy Chinese Adults.' *Nutrients* 14, 24 (2022): 5235. https://doi.org/10.3390/nu14245235

38. Slutsky, I., Abumaria, N., Wu, L.J., Huang, C., Zhang, L., Li, B., Zhao, X., Govindarajan, A., Zhao, M.G., Zhuo, M., Tonegawa, S., Liu, G., 'Enhancement of learning and memory by elevating brain magnesium.' *Neuron* 65, 2 (2010): 165–77. doi: 10.1016/j.neuron.2009.12.026

    Kim, Y.S., Won, Y.J., Lim, B.G., Min, T.J., Kim, Y.H., Lee, I.O., 'Neuroprotective effects of magnesium L-threonate in a hypoxic zebrafish model.' *BMC Neuroscience* 21, 1 (2020): 29. doi: 10.1186/s12868-020-00580-6

39. Vallée, A., Vallée, J.N., Lecarpentier, Y., 'Potential role of cannabidiol in Parkinson's disease by targeting the WNT/β-catenin pathway, oxidative stress and inflammation.' *Aging* 13, 7 (2021): 10796–10813. doi: 10.18632/aging.202951

Blessing, E.M., Steenkamp, M.M., Manzanares, J., Marmar, C.R., 'Cannabidiol as a Potential Treatment for Anxiety Disorders.' *Neurotherapeutics* 12, 4 (2015): 825–36. doi: 10.1007/s13311-015-0387-1

Bergamaschi, M.M., Queiroz, R,H., Zuardi, A.W., Crippa, J.A., 'Safety and side effects of cannabidiol, a Cannabis sativa constituent.' *Current Drug Safety* 6, 4 (2011): 237–49. doi: 10.2174/157488611798280924

Lee, S-H., et al, 'Multiple Forms of Endocannabinoid and Endovanilloid Signaling Regulate the Tonic Control of *GABA* Release.' *The Journal of Neuroscience* 35, 27 (2015): 10039–57. https://doi.org/10.1523/JNEUROSCI.4112-14.2015

40. Ranum, R.M., Whipple, M.O., Croghan, I., Bauer, B., Toussaint, L.L., Vincent, A., 'Use of Cannabidiol in the Management of Insomnia: A Systematic Review.' *Cannabis and Cannabinoid Research* 8, 2 (2023): 213–29. doi: 10.1089/can.2022.0122

Shannon, S., Lewis, N., Lee, H., Hughes, S., 'Cannabidiol in Anxiety and Sleep: A Large Case Series.' *The Permanente Journal* 23 (2019): 18–41. doi: 10.7812/*TPP*/18-041

41. Vigil, J.M., Stith, S.S., Diviant, J.P., Brockelman, F., Keeling, K., Hall, B., 'Effectiveness of Raw, Natural Medical Cannabis Flower for Treating Insomnia under Naturalistic Conditions.' *Medicines (Basel)* 5, 3 (2018): 75.

42. Suraev, A.S., Marshall, N.S., Vandrey, R., McCartney, D., Benson, M.J., McGregor, I.S., Grunstein, R.R., Hoyos, C.M., 'Cannabinoid therapies in the management of sleep disorders: A systematic review of preclinical and clinical studies.' *Sleep Medicine Reviews* 53 (2020): 101339. doi: 10.1016/j.smrv.2020.101339

Kaul, M., Zee, P.C., Sahni, A.S., 'Effects of Cannabinoids on Sleep and their Therapeutic Potential for Sleep Disorders.' *Neurotherapeutics* 18 (2021): 217–227. https://doi.org/10.1007/s13311-021-01013-w

Maddison, K.J., Kosky, C., Walsh, J.H., 'Is There a Place for Medicinal Cannabis in Treating Patients with Sleep Disorders? What We Know so Far.' *Nature and Science of Sleep* 14 (2022): 957–68. https://doi.org/10.2147/*NSS*.S340949

43. Gao, Q., Kou, T., Zhuang, B., Ren, Y., Dong, X., Wang, Q., 'The Association between Vitamin D Deficiency and Sleep Disorders: A Systematic Review and Meta-Analysis.' *Nutrients* 10, 10 (2018): 1395. doi: 10.3390/nu10101395

44. Abboud, M., 'Vitamin D Supplementation and Sleep: A Systematic Review and Meta-Analysis of Intervention Studies.' *Nutrients* 14 (2022): 1076. https://doi.org/10.3390/nu14051076

Romano, F., et al., 'Vitamin D and sleep regulation: is there a role for vitamin D?' *Current Pharmaceutical Design* 26 (2020): 2492–6. doi: 10.2174/1381 612826666200310145935

Muscogiuri, G., Barrea, L., Scannapieco, M., Di Somma, C., Scacchi, M., Aimaretti, G., et al., 'The lullaby of the sun: the role of vitamin D in sleep disturbance.' *Sleep Medicine* 54 (2019): 262–5. doi: 10.1016/j.sleep.2018.10.033

Al-Shawwa, B., Ehsan, Z., Ingram, D.G., 'Vitamin D and sleep in children.' *Journal of Clinical Sleep Medicine* 16 (2020): 1119–23. doi: 10.5664/jcsm.8440

45. 'New review launched into vitamin D intake to help tackle health disparities.' *Department of Health and Social Care* (3 April 2022). https://www.gov.uk/government/news/new-review-launched-into-vitamin-d-intake-to-help-tackle-health-disparities

Holick, M.F., 'The vitamin D deficiency pandemic: Approaches for diagnosis, treatment and prevention.' *Reviews in Endocrine and Metabolic Disorders* 18 (2017): 153–65. doi: 10.1007/s11154-017-9424-1

'Vitamin D: supplement use in specific population groups.' *NICE public health guidelines (PH56)* (26 November 2014, updated 30 August 2017). https://www.nice.org.uk/guidance/ph56

46. Swanson, C.M., Kohrt, W.M., Buxton, O.M., et al., 'The importance of the circadian system and sleep for bone health.' *Metabolism* 84 (2018): 28–43.

47. Ochs-Balcom, H.M., Hovey, K.M., Andrews, C., Cauley, J.A., Hale, L., Li, W., Bea, J.W., Sarto, G.E., Stefanick, M.L., Stone, K.L., Watts, N.B., Zaslavsky, O., Wactawski-Wende, J., 'Short Sleep Is Associated With Low Bone Mineral Density and Osteoporosis in the Women's Health Initiative.' *Journal of Bone and Mineral Research* 35, 2 (2020): 261–8. doi: 10.1002/jbmr.3879

'Bone Care for the Postmenopausal Woman.' *International Osteoporosis Foundation* (2013). http://share.iofbonehealth.org/WOD/2013/thematic-report/WOD13-Report.pdf.

48. Rosinger, A.Y., Chang, A.M., Buxton, O.M., Li, J., Wu, S., Gao, X., 'Short sleep duration is associated with inadequate hydration: Cross-cultural evidence from US and Chinese adults.' *Sleep* 42, 2 (2019). doi:10.1093/sleep/zsy210

Weissenberg, S., 'Insensible water loss during sleep: a theoretical exercise.' *Advances in Physiology Education* 29, 4 (2005): 213–15. https://www.physiology.org/doi/10.1152/advan.00028.2005

Dmitrieva, N.S., Burg, M.B., 'Increased insensible water loss contributes to aging related dehydration.' *PloS One* 6, 5 (2011): e20691.

Colwell, C.S., 'Preventing dehydration during sleep.' *Nature Neuroscience* 13, 4 (2010): 403–4. http://www.nature.com/articles/nn0410-403

49. Helaakoski, V., Kaprio, J., Hublin, C., Ollila, H.M., Latvala, A., 'Alcohol use and poor sleep quality: a longitudinal twin study across 36 years.' *SLEEP Advances* 3, 1 (2022). https://doi.org/10.1093/sleepadvances/zpac023

Ebrahim, I., Fenwick, P., Williams, A.J., Shapiro, C., 'Alcohol and sleep review: sound statistics and valid conclusions.' *Alcoholism: Clinical and Experimental Research* 39, 5 (2015): 944–6. doi: 10.1111/acer.12708

50. Einöther, S.J., Giesbrecht, T., 'Caffeine as an attention enhancer: reviewing existing assumptions.' *Psychopharmacology* 225, 2 (2013): 251–74.

Aidman, E., Balin, M., Johnson, K., et al., 'Caffeine may disrupt the impact of real-time drowsiness on cognitive performance: a double-blind, placebo-controlled small-sample study.' *Scientific Reports* 11, 4027 (2021). https://doi.org/10.1038/s41598-021-83504-6

Sherman, S.M., Buckley, T.P., Baena, E., Ryan, L., 'Caffeine Enhances Memory Performance in Young Adults during Their Non-optimal Time of Day.' *Frontiers in Psychology* 7 (2016): 1764. doi: 10.3389/fpsyg.2016.01764

51. O'Callaghan, F., Muurlink, O., Reid, N., 'Effects of caffeine on sleep quality and daytime functioning.' *Risk Management and Healthcare Policy* 11 (2018): 263–71. doi: 10.2147/RMHP.S156404

Blanchard, J., Sawers, S.J. 'The absolute bioavailability of caffeine in man.' *European Journal of Clinical Pharmacology* 24, 1 (1983): 93–8.

Snel, J., Lorist, M.M., 'Effects of caffeine on sleep and cognition.' *Progress in Brain Research* 190 (2011): 105–17.

Guest, N.S., VanDusseldorp, T.A., Nelson, M.T., et al., 'International society of sports nutrition position stand: caffeine and exercise performance.' *Journal of the International Society of Sports Nutrition* 18, 1 (2021). https://doi.org/10.1186/s12970-020-00383-4

52. Polasek, T.M., Patel, F., Jensen, B.P., Sorich, M.J., Wiese, M.D., Doogue, M.P., 'Predicted metabolic drug clearance with increasing adult age.' *British Journal of Clinical Pharmacology* 75, 4 (2013): 1019–28. doi: 10.1111/j.1365-2125.2012.04446.x

Drake, C., Roehrs, T., Shambroom, J., Roth, T., 'Caffeine effects on sleep taken 0, 3, or 6 hours before going to bed.' *Journal of Clinical Sleep Medicine* 9, 11 (2013): 1195–200. doi: 10.5664/jcsm.3170

53. Reichert, C.F., Deboer, T., Landolt, H.P., 'Adenosine, caffeine, and sleep-wake regulation: state of the science and perspectives.' *Journal of Sleep Research* 31, 4 (2022): e13597. doi: 10.1111/jsr.13597

Roehrs, T., Roth, T., 'Caffeine: sleep and daytime sleepiness.' *Sleep Medicine Reviews* 12 (2008): 153–62.

54. Burke, T.M., Markwald, R.R., McHill, A.W., Chinoy, E.D., Snider, J.A., Bessman, S.C., Jung, C.M., O'Neill, J.S., Wright, K.P. Jr., 'Effects of caffeine on the human circadian clock in vivo and in vitro.' *Science Translational Medicine* 7, 305 (2015): 305ra146. doi: 10.1126/scitranslmed.aac5125

55. Shilo, L., Sabbah, H., Hadari, R., et al., 'The effects of coffee consumption on sleep and melatonin secretion.' *Sleep Medicine* 3, 3 (2002): 271–3.

Snel, J., Lorist, M.M., 'Effects of caffeine on sleep and cognition.' *Progress in Brain Research* 190 (2011): 105–17.

Landolt, H.P., Werth, E., Borbély, A.A., Dijk, D.J., 'Caffeine intake (200 mg) in the morning affects human sleep and *EEG* power spectra at night.' *Brain Research* 675, 1–2 (1995): 67–74.

Kaplan, G.B., Greenblatt, D.J., Leduc, B.W., Thompson, M.L., Shader, R.I., 'Relationship of plasma and brain concentrations of caffeine and metabolites to benzodiazepine receptor binding and locomotor activity.' *Journal of Pharmacology and Experimental Therapeutics* 248, 3 (1989): 1078–83.

56. Naghma, K., Hasan, M., 'Tea and Health: Studies in Humans.' *Current Pharmaceutical Design* 19, 34 (2013). https://dx.doi.org/10.2174/13816128113193 40008

57. 'Caffeine.' *European Food Safety Authority.* https://www.efsa.europa.eu/en/topics/topic/caffeine

Reyes, C.M., Cornelis, M.C., 'Caffeine in the Diet: Country-Level Consumption and Guidelines.' *Nutrients* 10, 11 (2018): 1772. doi: 10.3390/nu10111772

Richards, G., Smith, A.P., 'A Review of Energy Drinks and Mental Health, with a Focus on Stress, Anxiety, and Depression.' *Journal of Caffeine Research* (2016): 49–63. https://doi.org/10.1089/jcr.2015.0033

58. Chang, S.M., Chen, C.H., 'Effects of an intervention with drinking chamomile tea on sleep quality and depression in sleep disturbed postnatal women: a randomized controlled trial.' *Journal of Advanced Nursing* 72, 2 (2016): 306–15. doi: 10.1111/jan.12836

Rafraf, M., Zemestani, M., Asghari-Jafarabadi, M., 'Effectiveness of chamomile tea on glycemic control and serum lipid profile in patients with type 2 diabetes.' *Journal of Endocrinological Investigation* 38, 2 (2015): 163–70. doi: 10.1007/s40618-014-0170-x

59. 'Satchidananda Panda, PhD.' *Salk Instiute for Biological Sciences.* https://www.salk.edu/scientist/satchidananda-panda/

60. 'Professor Tim Spector.' *King's College London.* https://www.kcl.ac.uk/people/professor-tim-spector

61. Simon, S.L., Blankenship, J., Manoogian, E.N.C., Panda, S., Mashek, D.G., Chow, L.S., 'The impact of a self-selected time restricted eating intervention on eating patterns, sleep, and late-night eating in individuals with obesity.' *Frontiers in Nutrition* 9 (2022). doi: 10.3389/fnut.2022.1007824

62. Wilkinson, M.J., Manoogian, E.N.C., Zadourian, A., Lo, H., Fakhouri, S., Shoghi, A., et al., 'Ten-hour time-restricted eating reduces weight, blood

pressure, and atherogenic lipids in patients with metabolic syndrome.' *Cell Metabolism* 31 (2020): 92–104. doi: 10.1016/j.cmet.2019.11.004

Lowe, D.A., Wu, N., Rohdin-Bibby, L., Moore, A.H., Kelly, N., Liu, Y.E., et al., 'Effects of time-restricted eating on weight loss and other metabolic parameters in women and men with overweight and obesity: the *TREAT* randomized clinical trial.' *JAMA Internal Medicine* 180 (2020): 1491–9. doi: 10.1001/jamainternmed.2020.4153

St-Onge, M.P., Ard, J., Baskin, M.L., Chiuve, S.E., Johnson, H.M., Kris-Etherton, P., et al., 'Meal timing and frequency: implications for cardiovascular disease prevention: a scientific statement from the American Heart Association.' *Circulation* 135 (2017): e96–e121. doi: 10.1161/CIR.0000000000000476

Yoshida, J., Eguchi, E., Nagaoka, K., Ito, T., Ogino, K., 'Association of night eating habits with metabolic syndrome and its components: a longitudinal study.' *BMC Public Health* 18 (2018): 1366. doi: 10.1186/s12889-018-6262-3

63. Manoogian, E.N.C., Chow, L.S., Taub, P.R., Laferrère, B., Panda, S., 'Time-restricted Eating for the Prevention and Management of Metabolic Diseases.' *Endocrine Reviews* 43, 2 (2022): 405–36. https://doi.org/10.1210/endrev/bnab027

Gill, S., Panda, S., 'A smartphone app reveals erratic diurnal eating patterns in humans that can be modulated for health benefits.' *Cell Metabolism* 22 (2015): 789–98. doi: 10.1016/j.cmet.2015.09.005

64. Smith, R.P., Easson, C., Lyle, S.M., Kapoor, R., Donnelly, C.P., Davidson, E.J., et al., 'Gut microbiome diversity is associated with sleep physiology in humans.' *PLoS One* 14, 10 (2019): e0222394. https://doi.org/10.1371/journal.pone.0222394

65. Smith, R.P., Easson, C., Lyle, S.M., Kapoor, R., Donnelly, C.P., Davidson, E.J., Parikh, E., Lopez, J.V., Tartar, J.L., 'Gut microbiome diversity is associated with sleep physiology in humans.' *PLoS One* 14, 10 (2019): e0222394. doi: 10.1371/journal.pone.0222394

66. Smith, R.P., Easson, C., Lyle, S.M., Kapoor, R., Donnelly, C.P., Davidson, E.J., Parikh, E., Lopez, J.V., Tartar, J.L., 'Gut microbiome diversity is associated with sleep physiology in humans.' *PLoS One* 14, 10 (2019): e0222394. doi: 10.1371/journal.pone.0222394

67. Sasso, J., Ammar, R.M., Tenchov R., Lemmel, S., Kelber, O., Grieswelle, M., Zhou, Q.A., 'Gut Microbiome–Brain Alliance: A Landscape View into Mental and Gastrointestinal Health and Disorders.' *ACS Chemical Neuroscience* 14, 10 (2023): 1717–63. https://doi.org/10.1021/acschemneuro.3c00127

68. Ogawa, Y., Miyoshi, C., Obana, N., et al., 'Gut microbiota depletion by chronic antibiotic treatment alters the sleep/wake architecture and sleep EEG power

spectra in mice.' *Scientific Reports* 10 (2020): 19554. https://doi.org/10.1038/s41598-020-76562-9

69. Benedict, C., Vogel, H., Jonas, W., Woting, A., Blaut, M., Schürmann, A., Cedernaes, J., 'Gut microbiota and glucometabolic alterations in response to recurrent partial sleep deprivation in normal-weight young individuals.' *Molecular Metabolism* 5, 12 (2016): 1175–86. https://doi.org/10.1016/j.molmet.2016.10.003

Withrow, D., Bowers, S.J., Depner, C.M., González, A., Reynolds, A.C., Wright, K.P. Jr., 'Sleep and Circadian Disruption and the Gut Microbiome-Possible Links to Dysregulated Metabolism.' *Current Opinion in Endocrine and Metabolic Research* 17 (2021): 26–37. doi: 10.1016/j.coemr.2020.11.009

Reynolds, A.C., Broussard, J., Paterson, J.L., Wright Jr., K.P., Ferguson, S.A., 'Sleepy, circadian disrupted and sick: Could intestinal microbiota play an important role in shift worker health?' *Molecular Metabolism* 6, 1 (2017): 12–13. https://doi.org/10.1016/j.molmet.2016.11.004

Krueger, J.M., Opp, M.R., 'Sleep and Microbes.' *International Review of Neurobiology* 131 (2016): 207–25. https://doi.org/10.1016/bs.irn.2016.07.003

Zhang, S.L., Bai, L., Goel, N., Bailey, A., Jang, C.J., Bushman, F.D., et al., 'Human and rat gut microbiome composition is maintained following sleep restriction.' *Proceedings of the National Academy of Sciences of the United States of America.* 114, 8 (2017): E1564–E71. doi:10.1073/pnas.1

70. Khanijow, V., Prakash, P., Emsellem, H.A., Borum, M.L., Doman, D.B., 'Sleep Dysfunction and Gastrointestinal Diseases.' *Gastroenterology & Hepatology* 11, 12 (2015): 817–25.

Smith, R.P., Easson, C., Lyle, S.M., Kapoor, R., Donnelly, C.P., Davidson, E.J., Parikh, E., Lopez, J.V., Tartar, J.L., 'Gut microbiome diversity is associated with sleep physiology in humans.' *PLoS One* 14, 10 (2019): e0222394. doi: 10.1371/journal.pone.0222394

71. Shaker, R., Castell, D.O., Schoenfeld, P.S., Spechler, S.J., 'Nighttime heartburn is an under-appreciated clinical problem that impacts sleep and daytime function: the results of a Gallup survey conducted on behalf of the American Gastroenterological Association.' *The American Journal of Gastroenterology* 98, 7 (2003): 1487–93.

Furukawa, Y., Cook, I.J., Panagopoulos, V., McEvoy, R.D., Sharp, D.J., Simula, M., 'Relationship between sleep patterns and human colonic motor patterns.' *Gastroenterology* 107, 5 (1994): 1372–81.

Saha, L., Malhotra, S., Rana, S., Bhasin, D., Pandhi, P., 'A preliminary study of melatonin in irritable bowel syndrome.' *Journal of Clinical Gastroenterology* 41, 1 (2007): 29–32.

Week 4: Combating Sleep Stress

1. De Nys, L., Anderson, K., Ofosu, E.F., Ryde, G.C., Connelly, J., Whittaker, A.C., 'The effects of physical activity on cortisol and sleep: A systematic review and meta-analysis.' *Psychoneuroendocrinology* 143 (2022). doi: 10.1016/j.psyneuen.2022.105843

   Buckley, T.M., Schatzberg, A.F., 'On the Interactions of the Hypothalamic-Pituitary-Adrenal (*HPA*) Axis and Sleep: Normal *HPA* Axis Activity and Circadian Rhythm, Exemplary Sleep Disorders.' *The Journal of Clinical Endocrinology & Metabolism* 90, 5 (2005): 3106–14. https://doi.org/10.1210/jc.2004-1056

2. Spiegel, K., Leproult, R., Van Cauter, E., 'Impact of sleep debt on metabolic and endocrine function.' *Lancet* 354 (1999): 1435–9.

   Buckley, T.M., Schatzberg, A.F., 'On the interactions of the hypothalamic-pituitary-adrenal (HPA) axis and sleep: normal HPA axis activity and circadian rhythm, exemplary sleep disorders.' *The Journal of Clinical Endocrinology and Metabolism* 90, 5 (2005): 3106–14.

   Spath-Schwalbe, E., Scholler, T., Kern, W., Fehm, H.L., Born, J., 'Nocturnal adrenocorticotropin and cortisol secretion depends on sleep duration and decreases in association with spontaneous awakening in the morning.' *The Journal of Clinical Endocrinology and Metabolism* 75, 6 (1992): 1431–5.

   Hirotsu, C., Tufik, S., Andersen, M.L., 'Interactions between sleep, stress, and metabolism: From physiological to pathological conditions.' *Sleep Science* 8, 3 (2015): 143–52. doi: 10.1016/j.slsci.2015.09.002

3. 'Stress and sleep', *American Psychological Association* (1 January 2013). https://www.apa.org/news/press/releases/stress/2013/sleep

   Chattu, V.K., Manzar, M.D., Kumary, S., Burman, D., Spence, D.W., Pandi-Perumal, S.R., 'The Global Problem of Insufficient Sleep and Its Serious Public Health Implications.' *Healthcare (Basel)* 7, 1 (2018): 1. doi: 10.3390/healthcare7010001

   Åkerstedt, T., Orsini, N., Petersen, H., 'Predicting sleep quality from stress and prior sleep–a study of day-to-day covariation across six weeks.' *Sleep Medicine* 13, 6 (2012): 674–9.

   Eliasson, A.H., Kashani, M., Mayhew, M., 'Reducing perceived stress improves sleep quality: a longitudinal outcomes study.' *Chest* 138, 4 (2010): 913A. doi: 10.1378/chest

   Kim, H.J., Oh, S.Y., Joo, J.H., Choi, D.-W., Park, E.-C., 'The Relationship between Sleep Duration and Perceived Stress: Findings from the 2017 Community Health Survey in Korea.' *International Journal of Environmental Research and Public Health* 16 (2019). https://doi.org/10.3390/ijerph16173208

4. Mohd Azmi, N.A.S., Juliana, N., Azmani, S., Mohd Effendy, N., Abu, I.F., Mohd Fahmi Teng, N.I., Das, S., 'Cortisol on Circadian Rhythm and Its

Effect on Cardiovascular System.' International *Journal of Environmental Research and Public Health* 18, 2 (2021): 676. doi: 10.3390/ijerph18020676

Hirotsu, C., Tufik, S., Andersen, M.L., 'Interactions between sleep, stress, and metabolism: From physiological to pathological conditions.' *Sleep Science* 8, 3 (2015): 143–52. doi: 10.1016/j.slsci.2015.09.002

Zisapel, N., 'New Perspectives on the Role of Melatonin in Human Sleep, Circadian Rhythms and Their Regulation.' *British Journal of Pharmacology* 175, 16 (2018): 3190–9.

5. Maki, P.M., Mordecai, K.L., Rubin, L.H., Sundermann, E., Savarese, A., Eatough, E., Drogos, L., 'Menstrual cycle effects on cortisol responsivity and emotional retrieval following a psychosocial stressor.' *Hormones and Behavior* 74 (2015): 201–8. doi: 10.1016/j.yhbeh.2015.06.023

Zisapel, N., 'New perspectives on the role of melatonin in human sleep, circadian rhythms and their regulation.' *British Journal of Pharmacology* 175 16 (2018): 3190–9. doi: 10.1111/bph.14116

Chen, J., 'Women, Are Your Hormones Keeping You up at Night?' *Yale Medicine* (10 July 2017), www.yalemedicine.org/news/women-are-your-hormones-keeping-you-up-at-night

6. Kim, T.W., Jeong, J.H. and Hong, S.C., 'The impact of sleep and circadian disturbance on hormones and metabolism.' *International Journal of Endocrinology* (2015). doi: 10.1155/2015/591729

Lee, J., Han, Y., Cho, H.H., Kim, M.R., 'Sleep Disorders and Menopause.' *Journal of Menopausal Medicine* 25, 2 (2019): 83–7. https://pubmed.ncbi.nlm.nih.gov/31497577/

Joffe, H., Massler, A., Sharkey, K.M., 'Evaluation and management of sleep disturbance during the menopause transition.' *Seminars in Reproductive Medicine* 28, 5 (2010): 404–21. https://pubmed.ncbi.nlm.nih.gov/20845239/

Mirer, A.G., Young, T., Palta, M., Benca, R.M., Rasmuson, A., Peppard, P.E., 'Sleep-disordered breathing and the menopausal transition among participants in the Sleep in Midlife Women Study.' *Menopause* 24, 2 (2017): 157–62. https://pubmed.ncbi.nlm.nih.gov/27760083/

Baker, F.C., et al., 'Sleep problems during the menopausal transition: prevalence, impact, and management challenges.' *Nature and Science of Sleep* 10 (2018): 73–95. doi: 10.2147/NSS.S125807

7. Reed, S.D., Newton, K.M., Larson, J.C., Booth-LaForce, C., Woods, N.F., Landis, C.A., Tolentino, E., Carpenter, J.S., Freeman, E.W., Joffe, H., Anawalt, B.D., Guthrie, K.A., 'Daily salivary cortisol patterns in midlife women with hot flashes.' *Clinical Endocrinology* 84, 5 (2016): 672–9. doi: 10.1111/cen.12995

Woods, N.F., Mitchell, E.S., Smith-Dijulio, K., 'Cortisol levels during the menopausal transition and early postmenopause: observations from the Seattle Midlife Women's Health Study.' *Menopause* 16, 4 (2009): 708–18. doi: 10.1097/gme.0b013e318198d6b2

Gerber, L.M., Sievert, L.L., Schwartz, J.E., 'Hot flashes and midlife symptoms in relation to levels of salivary cortisol.' *Maturitas* 96 (2017): 26–32. doi: 10.1016/j.maturitas.2016.11.001

8. Jungmann, M., Vencatachellum, S., Van Ryckeghem, D., Vögele, C., 'Effects of Cold Stimulation on Cardiac-Vagal Activation in Healthy Participants: Randomized Controlled Trial.' *JMIR Formative Research* 2, 2 (2018): e10257. doi: 10.2196/10257

Pigarev, I.N., Pigareva, M.L., Levichkina, E.V., 'Probable Mechanism of Antiepileptic Effect of the Vagus Nerve Stimulation in the Context of the Recent Results in Sleep Research.' *Frontiers in Neuroscience* 14 (2020): 160. doi: 10.3389/fnins.2020.00160

9. Moore, E., Fuller, J.T., Bellenger, C.R., et al., 'Effects of Cold-Water Immersion Compared with Other Recovery Modalities on Athletic Performance Following Acute Strenuous Exercise in Physically Active Participants: A Systematic Review, Meta-Analysis, and Meta-Regression.' *Sports Medicine* 53 (2023): 687–705. https://doi.org/10.1007/s40279-022-01800-1

Leeder, J., Gissane, C., van Someren, K., Gregson, W., Howatson, G., 'Cold water immersion and recovery from strenuous exercise: a meta-analysis.' *British Journal of Sports Medicine* 46 (2012): 233–40. doi: 10.1136/bjsports-2011-090061

Allan, R., Malone, J., Alexander, J., et al., 'Cold for centuries: a brief history of cryotherapies to improve health, injury and post-exercise recovery.' *European Journal of Appled Physiology* 122 (2022): 1153–62. https://doi.org/10.1007/s00421-022-04915-5

10. Chan, S.H.M., Qiu, L., Esposito, G., et al., 'Nature in virtual reality improves mood and reduces stress: evidence from young adults and senior citizens.' *Virtual Reality* (2021). https://doi.org/10.1007/s10055-021-00604-4

11. Wood, A.M., Joseph, S., Lloyd, J., Atkins, S., 'Gratitude influences sleep through the mechanism of pre-sleep cognitions.' *Journal of Psychosomatic Research* 66, 1 (2009): 43–8. doi: 10.1016/j.jpsychores.2008.09.002

12. Zahn, R., Moll, J., Paiva, M., Garrido, G., Krueger, F., Huey, E.D., Grafman, J., 'The neural basis of human social values: evidence from functional MRI.' *Cerebral Cortex* 19, 2 (2009): 276–83. doi: 10.1093/cercor/bhn080

Seligman, M.E., Steen, T.A., Park, N., Peterson, C., 'Positive psychology progress: empirical validation of interventions.' *American Psychologist* 60, 5 (2005): 410–21. doi: 10.1037/0003-066X.60.5.410

13. Kyeong, S., Kim, J., Kim, D., et al., 'Effects of gratitude meditation on neural network functional connectivity and brain-heart coupling.' *Scientific Reports* 7, 5058 (2017). https://doi.org/10.1038/s41598-017-05520-9

14. Jackowska, M., et al., 'The impact of a brief gratitude intervention on subjective well-being, biology and sleep.' *Journal of Health Psychology* 21, 10 (2016): 2207–17.

15. Wood, A.M, Joseph, S., Lloyd, J., Atkins, S., 'Gratitude influences sleep through the mechanism of pre-sleep cognitions.' *Journal of Psychosomatic Research* 66 (2009): 43–8. doi: 10.1016/j.jpsychores.2008.09.002

16. Wood, A.M., Joseph, S., Lloyd, J., Atkins, S., 'Gratitude influences sleep through the mechanism of pre-sleep cognitions.' *Journal of Psychosomatic Research* 66, 1 (2009): 43–8. doi: 10.1016/j.jpsychores.2008.09.002

    Zahn, R., Moll, J., Paiva, M., Garrido, G., Krueger, F., Huey, E.D., Grafman, J., 'The neural basis of human social values: evidence from functional MRI.' *Cerebral Cortex* 19, 2 (2009): 276–83. doi: 10.1093/cercor/bhn080

    Wong, Y.J., Owen, J., Gabana, N.T., Brown, J.W., McInnis, S., Toth P., Gilman, L., 'Does gratitude writing improve the mental health of psychotherapy clients? Evidence from a randomized controlled trial.' *Psychotherapy Research* 28, 2 (2018): 192–202. doi: 10.1080/10503307.2016.1169332

    Garland, S.N., Carlson, L.E., et al., 'Mindfulness-based stress reduction compared with cognitive behavioral therapy for the treatment of insomnia comorbid with cancer: a randomized, partially blinded, noninferiority trial.' *Journal of Clinical Oncology* 32, 5 (2014): 449–57.

    Goldin, P.R., Gross, J.J., 'Effects of mindfulness-based stress reduction (MBSR) on emotion regulation in social anxiety disorder.' *Emotion* 10, 1 (2010): 83–91.

17. Wood, A.M., Joseph, S., Lloyd, J., Atkins, S., 'Gratitude influences sleep through the mechanism of pre-sleep cognitions.' *Journal of Psychosomatic Research* 66, 1 (2009): 43–8. doi: 10.1016/j.jpsychores.2008.09.002

18. Fox, G.R., Kaplan, J., Damasio, H., Damasio, A., 'Neural correlates of gratitude.' *Frontiers in Psychology* 6 (2015): 1491. doi: 10.3389/fpsyg.2015.01491

    Cunha, L.F., Pellanda, L.C., Reppold, C.T., 'Positive Psychology and Gratitude Interventions: A Randomized Clinical Trial.' *Frontiers in Psychology* 10 (2019): 584. doi: 10.3389/fpsyg.2019.00584

19. Fox, G.R., Kaplan, J., Damasio, H., Damasio, A., 'Neural correlates of gratitude.' *Frontiers in Psychology* 6 (2015). doi: 10.3389/fpsyg.2015.01491

    Zahn, R., Moll, J., Paiva, M., Garrido, G., Krueger, F., Huey, E.D., Grafman, J., 'The Neural Basis of Human Social Values: Evidence from Functional MRI.' *Cerebral Cortex* 19, 2 (2009): 276–83. https://doi.org/10.1093/cercor/bhn080

20. Scullin, M.K., Krueger, M.L., Ballard, H.K., Pruett, N., Bliwise, D.L., 'The effects of bedtime writing on difficulty falling asleep: A polysomnographic study comparing to-do lists and completed activity lists.' *Journal of Experimental Psychology: General* 147, 1 (2018): 139–46. doi: 10.1037/xge0000374

Alkozei, A., Smith, R., Kotzin, M.D., Waugaman, D.L., Killgore, W.D.S., 'The Association Between Trait Gratitude and Self-Reported Sleep Quality Is Mediated by Depressive Mood State.' *Behavioral Sleep Medicine* 17, 1 (2019): 41–8. doi: 10.1080/15402002.2016.1276017

21. Harmat, L., Takács, J., Bódizs, R., 'Music improves sleep quality in students.' *Journal of Advanced Nursing* 62, 3 (2008): 327–35. doi: 10.1111/j.1365-2648.2008.04602.x

Cordi, M.J., Ackermann, S., Rasch, B., 'Effects of Relaxing Music on Healthy Sleep.' *Scientific Reports* 9 (2019). https://doi.org/10.1038/s41598-019-45608-y

22. Gould van Praag, C.D., Garfinkel, S.N., Sparasci, O., Mees, A., Philippides, A.O., Ware, M., Ottaviani, C., Critchley, H.D., 'Mind-wandering and alterations to default mode network connectivity when listening to naturalistic versus artificial sounds.' *Scientific Reports* 7 (2017). doi: 10.1038/srep45273

23. Koulivand, P.H., Khaleghi Ghadiri, M., Gorji, A., 'Lavender and the nervous system.' *Evidence-Based Complementary and Alternative Medicine* (2013): 681304. doi: 10.1155/2013/681304

Braden, R., Reichow, S., Halm, M.A., 'The use of the essential oil lavandin to reduce preoperative anxiety in surgical patients.' *Journal of PeriAnesthesia Nursing* 24, 6 (2009): 348–55. doi: 10.1016/j.jopan.2009.10.002

24. McKeown, P., O'Connor-Reina, C., Plaza, G., 'Breathing Re-Education and Phenotypes of Sleep Apnea: A Review.' *Journal of Clinical Medicine* 10, 3 (2021): 471. doi: 10.3390/jcm10030471

25. Seppälä, E.J., Nitschke, J.B., Tudorascu, D.L., Hayes, A., Goldstein, M.R., Nguyen, D.T.H., Perlman, D., Davidson, R.J., 'Breathing-Based Meditation Decreases Posttraumatic Stress Disorder Symptoms in U.S. Military Veterans: A Randomized Controlled Longitudinal Study.' *Journal of Traumatic Stress* 27, 4 (2014): 397–405. https://doi.org/10.1002/jts.21936

26. Jerath, R., Beveridge, C., Barnes, V.A., 'Self-regulation of breathing as an adjunctive treatment of insomnia.' *Front Psychiatry* 29, 9 (2019): 780. doi: 10.3389/fpsyt.2018.00780. PMID: 30761030; PMCID: PMC6361823.

Rusch, H.L., Rosario, M., Levison, L.M., Olivera, A., Livingston, W.S., Wu, T., Gill, J.M., 'The effect of mindfulness meditation on sleep quality: a systematic review and meta-analysis of randomized controlled trials.' *Annals of the New York Academy of Sciences* 1445 (2019): 5–16. https://doi.org/10.1111/nyas.13996

27. Laborde, S., Hosang, T., Mosley, E., Dosseville, F., 'Influence of a 30-Day Slow-Paced Breathing Intervention Compared to Social Media Use on Subjective Sleep Quality and Cardiac Vagal Activity.' *Journal of Clinical Medicine* 8, 2 (2019): 193. https://doi.org/10.3390/jcm8020193

28. Philip, K.E.J., Owles, H., McVey, S., Pagnuco, T., Bruce, K., Brunjes, H., et al, 'An online breathing and wellbeing programme (ENO Breathe) for people with persistent symptoms following COVID-19: a parallel-group, single-blind, randomised controlled trial.' *The Lancet* 10, 9 (2022): 851–62. https://doi.org/10.1016/S2213-2600(22)00125-4

29. Su, H., Xiao, L., Ren, Y., Xie, H., Sun, X.H., 'Effects of mindful breathing combined with sleep-inducing exercises in patients with insomnia.' *World Journal of Clinical Cases* 9, 29 (2021): 8740–8 doi: https://dx.doi.org/10.12998/wjcc.v9.i29.8740

30. 'The Science of Gratitude and How to Build a Gratitude Practice.' *Huberman Lab* (22 November 2021), https://hubermanlab.com/the-science-of-gratitude-and-how-to-build-a-gratitude-practice/

31. Arshamian, A., Iravani, B., Majid A., Lundström, J.N., 'Respiration Modulates Olfactory Memory Consolidation in Humans.' *The Journal of Neuroscience* 38, 48 (2018): 10286–94. doi: https://doi.org/10.1523/JNEUROSCI.3360-17.2018

Week 5: The Importance of Regular Rest and Well-Timed Exercise for Sleep Health

1. Goleman, D., et al., *Focus (HBR Emotional Intelligence Series)* (Harvard Business Press, 2018).

2. Suda, M., et al., 'Subjective feeling of psychological fatigue is related to decreased reactivity in ventrolateral prefrontal cortex.' *Brain Research* 1252 (2009): 152–60.

   Alexander, N.B., et al., 'Bedside-to-bench conference: research agenda for idiopathic fatigue and aging.' *Journal of the American Geriatrics Society* 58, 5 (2010): 967–75.

   McMorris, T., et al., 'Cognitive fatigue effects on physical performance: A systematic review and meta-analysis.' *Physiology & Behavior* 188 (2018): 103–7.

3. Morita, E., Imai, M., Okawa, M., Miyaura, T., Miyazaki, S., 'A before and after comparison of the effects of forest walking on the sleep of a community-based sample of people with sleep complaints.' *BioPsychoSocial Medicine* 5, 13 (2011). doi: 10.1186/1751-0759-5-13

   Grigsby-Toussaint, D.S., Turi, K.N., Krupa, M., Williams, N.J., Pandi-Perumal, S.R., Jean-Louis, G., 'Sleep insufficiency and the natural environment:

Results from the US Behavioral Risk Factor Surveillance System Survey.' *Preventative Medicine* 78 (2015): 78–84. doi:10.1016/j.ypmed.2015.07.011

Ohly, H., White, M.P., Wheeler, B.W., Bethel, A., Ukoumunne, O.C., Nikolaou, V., Garside, R., 'Attention Restoration Theory: A systematic review of the attention restoration potential of exposure to natural environments.' *Journal of Toxicology and Environmental Health, Part B* 19, 7 (2016): 305–43. doi: 10.1080/10937404.2016.1196155

Gladwell, V.F., Kuoppa, P., Tarvainen, M.P., Rogerson, M., 'A Lunchtime Walk in Nature Enhances Restoration of Autonomic Control during Night-Time Sleep: Results from a Preliminary Study.' *International Journal of Environmental Research and Public Health* 13, 3 (2016): 280. https://doi.org/10.3390/ijerph13030280

4. Sullivan Bisson, A.N., Robinson, S.A., Lachman, M.E., 'Walk to a better night of sleep: testing the relationship between physical activity and sleep.' *Sleep Health* 5, 5 (2019): 487–94. doi: 10.1016/j.sleh.2019.06.003

5. Murray, K., Godbole, S., Natarajan, L., et al., 'The relations between sleep, time of physical activity, and time outdoors among adult women.' *PLoS One* 12, 9 (2017): e0182013. doi:10.1371/journal.pone.0182013

Moss, T.G., Carney, C.E., Haynes, P., Harris, A.L., 'Is daily routine important for sleep? An investigation of social rhythms in a clinical insomnia population.' *Chronobiology International* 32, 1 (2015): 92–102. doi:10.3109/07420528.2014.956361

6. Lovato, N., Lack, L., 'The effects of napping on cognitive functioning.' *Progress in Brain Research* 185 (2010): 155–66. doi: 10.1016/B978-0-444-53702-7.00009-9

Paz, V., Dashti, H.S., Garfield, V., 'Is there an association between daytime napping, cognitive function, and brain volume? A Mendelian randomization study in the UK Biobank.' *Sleep Health* (2023). https://doi.org/10.1016/j.sleh.2023.05.002

Souabni, M., Hammouda, O., Romdhani, M., Trabelsi, K., Ammar, A., Driss, T., 'Benefits of Daytime Napping Opportunity on Physical and Cognitive Performances in Physically Active Participants: A Systematic Review.' *Sports Medicine* 51, 10 (2021): 2115–46. doi: 10.1007/s40279-021-01482-1

7. Mesas, A.E., Núñez de Arenas-Arroyo, S., Martinez-Vizcaino, V., et al, 'Is daytime napping an effective strategy to improve sport-related cognitive and physical performance and reduce fatigue? A systematic review and meta-analysis of randomised controlled trials.' *British Journal of Sports Medicine* 57 (2023): 417–26.

8. Milner, C.E., Cote, K.A., 'Benefits of napping in healthy adults: impact of nap length, time of day, age, and experience with napping.' *Journal of Sleep Research* 18, 2 (2009): 272–81. doi: 10.1111/j.1365-2869.2008.00718.x

Goldschmied, J., et al., 'Napping to modulate frustration and impulsivity: A pilot study. Personality and Individual Differences.' *Personality and Individual Differences* 86 (2015): 164–7.

Mednick, S., Nakayama, K., Stickgold, R., 'Sleep-dependent learning: a nap is as good as a night.' *Nature Neuroscience* 6, 7 (2003): 697–8.

Whitehurst, L.N., et al., 'Autonomic activity during sleep predicts memory consolidation in humans.' *Proceedings of the National Academy of Sciences* 113, 26 (2016): 7272–7.

Mednick, S.C., Cai, D.J., Kanady, J., Drummond, S.P.A., 'Comparing the benefits of Caffeine, Naps and Placebo on Verbal, Motor and Perceptual Memory.' *Behavioral Brain Research* 193, 1 (2008): 79–86.

Hayashi, M., Masuda, A., Hori, T., 'The alerting effects of caffeine, bright light and face washing after a short daytime nap.' *Clinical Neurophysiology* 114, 12 (2003): 2268–78.

9. 'Physical activity; applying All Our Health.' *Gov.uk*, www.gov.uk/government/publications/physical-activity-applying-all-our-health/physical-activity-applying-all-our-health

10. Passos, G.S., Poyares, D.L, Santana, M.G., Tufik, S., Mello, M.T., 'Is exercise an alternative treatment for chronic insomnia?' *Clinics (Sao Paulo)* 67, 6 (2012): 653–60. doi: 10.6061/clinics/2012(06)17

    Kline, C.E., 'The bidirectional relationship between exercise and sleep: Implications for exercise adherence and sleep improvement.' *American Journal of Lifestyle Medicine* 8, 6 (2014): 375–9. doi: 10.1177/1559827614544437

11. Dolezal, B.A., Neufeld, E.V., Boland, D.M., Martin, J.L., Cooper, C.B., 'Interrelationship between sleep and exercise: a systematic review.' *Advances in Preventive Medicine* (2017): 14. doi: 10.1155/2017/1364387.1364387

    D'Aurea, C.V.R., Poyares, D., Passos, G.S., Santana, M.G., Youngstedt, S.D., Souza, A.A., Bicudo, J., Tufik, S., de Mello, M.T., 'Effects of resistance exercise training and stretching on chronic insomnia.' *Brazilian Journal of Psychiatry* 41, 1 (2018).

    Wang, F., Boros, S., 'The effect of physical activity on sleep quality: a systematic review.' *European Journal of Physiotherapy* 23, 1 (2021): 11–18. doi: 10.1080/21679169.2019.1623314

    Brupbacher, G., Straus, D., Porschke, H., et al., 'The acute effects of aerobic exercise on sleep in patients with depression: study protocol for a randomized controlled trial.' *Trials* 20, 352 (2019). https://doi.org/10.1186/s13063-019-3415-3

12. Alley, J.R., Mazzochi, J.W., Smith, C.J., Morris, D.M., Collier, S.R., 'Effects of resistance exercise timing on sleep architecture and nocturnal blood pressure.' *The Journal of Strength and Conditioning Research* 29, 5 (2015): 1378–85. doi: 10.1519/JSC.0000000000000750

Qian, J., Sun, S., Wang, M., Sun, Y., Sun, X., Jevitt, C., Yu, X., 'The effect of exercise intervention on improving sleep in menopausal women: a systematic review and meta-analysis.' *Frontiers in Medicine* 10 (2023). https://doi.org/10.3389/fmed.2023.1092294

Glavin, E.E., Ceneus, M., Chanowitz, M., Kantilierakis, J., Mendelow, E., Mosquera, J., Spaeth, A.M., 'Relationships between sleep, exercise timing, and chronotype in young adults.' *Journal of Health Psychology* 26, 13 (2021): 2636–47. doi: 10.1177/1359105320926530

13. Dolezal, B.A., Neufeld, E.V., Boland, D.M., Martin, J.L., Cooper, C.B., 'Interrelationship between Sleep and Exercise: A Systematic Review.' *Advances in Preventative Medicine* (2017). doi: 10.1155/2017/1364387

14. Villemure, C., Ceko, M., Cotton, V.A., Bushnell, M.C., 'Insular cortex mediates increased pain tolerance in yoga practitioners.' *Cerebral Cortex* 24, 10 (2014): 2732–40. doi: 10.1093/cercor/bht124

15. Kumar, V., Malhotra, V., Kumar, S., 'Application of Standardised Yoga Protocols as the Basis of Physiotherapy Recommendation in Treatment of Sleep Apneas: Moving Beyond Pranayamas.' *Indian Journal of Otolaryngology and Head and Neck Surgery* 71, Suppl 1 (2019): 558–65. doi: 10.1007/s12070-018-1405-5

16. Wang, W.L., Chen, K.H., Pan, Y.C., et al., 'The effect of yoga on sleep quality and insomnia in women with sleep problems: a systematic review and meta-analysis.' *BMC Psychiatry* 20, 195 (2020). https://doi.org/10.1186/s12888-020-02566-4

Vera, F.M., Manzaneque, J.M., Maldonado, E.F., Carranque, G.A., Rodriguez, F.M., Blanca, M.J., Morell, M., 'Subjective sleep quality and hormonal modulation in long-term yoga practitioners.' *Biological Psychology* 81, 3 (2009): 164–8. doi: 10.1016/j.biopsycho.2009.03.008

17. Chen, Z., Ye, X., Shen, Z., Chen, G., Chen, W., He, T., Xu, X., 'Effect of Pilates on Sleep Quality: A Systematic Review and Meta-Analysis of Randomized Controlled Trials.' *Frontiers in Neurology* 11 (2020): 158. doi: 10.3389/fneur.2020.00158

18. Caldwell, K., Harrison, M., Adams, M., Triplett, N.T., 'Effect of Pilates and Taiji Quan Training on Self-Efficacy, Sleep Quality, Mood, and Physical Performance of College Students.' *Journal of Bodywork and Movement Therapies* 13, 2 (2009): 155–63. https://doi.org/10.1016/j.jbmt.2007.12.001

19. Siu, P.M., Yu, A.P., Tam, B.T., Chin, E.C., Yu, D.S., Chung, K.F., Hui, S.S., Woo, J., Fong, D.Y., Lee, P.H., Wei, G.X., Irwin, M.R., 'Effects of Tai Chi or Exercise on Sleep in Older Adults With Insomnia: A Randomized Clinical Trial.' *JAMA Network Open* 4, 2 (2021): e2037199. doi: 10.1001/jamanetworkopen.2020.37199

20. Chauvineau, M., Pasquier, F., Guyot, V., Aloulou, A., Nedelec, M., 'Effect of the Depth of Cold Water Immersion on Sleep Architecture and Recovery Among Well-Trained Male Endurance Runners.' *Frontiers in Sports and Active Living* 3 (2021). doi: 10.3389/fspor.2021.659990

21. Demori, I., Piccinno, T., Saverino, D., et al., 'Effects of winter sea bathing on psychoneuroendocrinoimmunological parameters.' *Explore* 17, 2 (2021): 122–6.

Huttunen, P., Kokko, L., Ylijukuri, V., 'Winter swimming improves general well-being.' *International Journal of Circumpolar Health* 63, 2 (2004): 140–4.

22. Yankouskaya, A., Williamson, R., Stacey, C., Totman, J.J., Massey, H., 'Short-Term Head-Out Whole-Body Cold-Water Immersion Facilitates Positive Affect and Increases Interaction between Large-Scale Brain Networks.' *Biology* 12 (2023): 211. https://doi.org/10.3390/biology12020211

Vaswani, K.K., Richard, C.W. 3rd, Tejwani, G.A., 'Cold swim stress-induced changes in the levels of opioid peptides in the rat *CNS* and peripheral tissues.' *Pharmacology Biochemistry and Behavior* 29, 1 (1988): 163–8. doi: 10.1016/0091-3057(88)90290-0

Shevchuk, N.A., 'Adapted cold shower as a potential treatment for depression.' *Medical Hypotheses* 70, 5 (2008): 995–1001. https://doi.org/10.1016/j.mehy.2007.04.052

King, M., Carnahan, H., 'Revisiting the brain activity associated with innocuous and noxious cold exposure.' *Neuroscience and Biobehavioral Reviews* 104 (2019): 197–208. https://doi.org/10.1016/j.neubiorev.2019.06.021

Nédélec, M., Halson, S., Delecroix, B., Abaidia, A.E., Ahmaidi, S., Dupont, G., 'Sleep Hygiene and Recovery Strategies in Elite Soccer Players.' *Sports Medicine* 45, 11 (2015): 1547–59. doi: 10.1007/s40279-015-0377-9

23. Haghayegh, S., Khoshnevis, S., Smolensky, M.H., Diller, K.R., Castriotta, R.J., 'Before-bedtime passive body heating by warm shower or bath to improve sleep: A systematic review and meta-analysis.' *Sleep Medicine Reviews* 46 (2019): 124–35. https://pubmed.ncbi.nlm.nih.gov/31102877/

Tai, Y., Obayashi, K., Yamagami, Y., Yoshimoto, K., Kurumatani, N., Nishio, K., Saeki, K., 'Hot-water bathing before bedtime and shorter sleep onset latency are accompanied by a higher distal-proximal skin temperature gradient in older adults.' *Journal of Clinical Sleep Medicine* 17, 6 (2021): 1257–66.

Tai, Y., Saeki, K., Yamagami, Y., Yoshimoto, K., Kurumatani, N., Nishio, K., Obayashi, K., 'Association between timing of hot water bathing before bedtime and night-/sleep-time blood pressure and dipping in the elderly: A longitudinal analysis for repeated measurements in home settings.' *Chronobiology International* 36, 12 (2019): 1714–22.

Bleakley, C.M., Davison, G.W., 'What is the biochemical and physiological rationale for using cold-water immersion in sports recovery? A systematic review.' *British Journal of Sports Medicine* 44 (2010): 179–87. https://bjsm.bmj.com/content/44/3/179

Minett, G.M., Gale, R., Wingfield, G., Marino, F.E., Washington, T.L., Skein, M., 'Sleep quantity and quality during heat-based training and the effects of cold-water immersion recovery.' *Extreme Physiology and Medicine* 4, Suppl 1 (2015): 150–1.

Buijze, G.A., Sierevelt, I.N., van der Heijden, B.C.J.M., Dijkgraaf, M.G., Frings-Dresen, M.H.W., 'The effect of cold showering on health and work: A randomized controlled trial.' *PLoS One* 11, 9 (2016): e0161749. https://pubmed.ncbi.nlm.nih.gov/27631616/

24. Haghayegh, S., Khoshnevis, S., Smolensky, M.H., Diller, K.R., Castriotta, R.J., 'Before-bedtime passive body heating by warm shower or bath to improve sleep: A systematic review and meta-analysis.' *Sleep Medicine Reviews* 46 (2019): 124–35. doi: 10.1016/j.smrv.2019.04.008

25. Rafii, F., Ameri, F., Haghani, H., et al., 'The effect of aromatherapy massage with lavender and chamomile oil on anxiety and sleep quality of patients with burns.' *Burns* 46 (2020): 164–71.

Kim, M.E., Jun, J.H., Hur, M.H., 'Effects of aromatherapy on sleep quality: a systematic review and meta- analysis.' *Journal of Korean Academy of Nursing* 49 (2019): 655–76.

Hwang, E., Shin, S., 'The effects of aromatherapy on sleep improvement: a systematic literature review and meta-analysis.' *Journal of Alternative and Complementary Medicine* 21 (2015): 61–8.

Common Sleep Problems

1. Bhaskar, S., Hemavathy, D., Prasad, S., 'Prevalence of chronic insomnia in adult patients and its correlation with medical comorbidities.' *Journal of Family Medicine and Primary* Care 5, 4 (2016): 780–4. doi: 10.4103/2249-4863.201153

Riemann, D., Benz, F., Dressle, R.J., Espie, C.A., Johann, A.F., Blanken, T.F., Leerssen, J., Wassing, R., Henry, A.L., Kyle, S.D., et al., 'Insomnia disorder: State of the science and challenges for the future.' *Journal of Sleep Research* 31 (2022): e13604. doi: 10.1111/jsr.13604.

Léger, D., Bayon, V., 'Societal costs of insomnia.' *Sleep Medicine Reviews* 14, 6 (2010): 379–89.

Ohayon, M.M., Partinen, M., 'Insomnia and global sleep dissatisfaction in Finland.' *Journal of Sleep Research* 11, 4 (2002): 339–46.

2. Morphy, H., Dunn, K.M., Boardman, H.F., Croft, P.R., 'Epidemiology of insomnia: a longitudinal study in a UK population.' *Sleep* 30, 3 (2007), 274–80.

'How common is it?' *NICE* (May 2022), https://cks.nice.org.uk/topics/insomnia/background-information/prevalence/

'Insomnia.' *NICE Clinical Knowledge* (May 2022), https://cks.nice.org.uk/topics/insomnia/

3. Passos, G.S., Poyares, D.L., Santana, M.G., Tufik, S., Mello, M.T., 'Is exercise an alternative treatment for chronic insomnia?' *Clinics (Sao Paulo)* 67, 6 (2012): 653–60. doi: 10.6061/clinics/2012(06)17

   Hartescu, I., Morgan, K., Stevinson, C.D., 'Increased physical activity improves sleep and mood outcomes in inactive people with insomnia: a randomized controlled trial.' *Journal of Sleep Research* 24, 5 (2015): 526–34. https://doi.org/10.1111/jsr.12297

   Marcus, R.L., Lastayo, P.C., Dibble, L.E., Hill, L., McClain, D.A., 'Increased strength and physical performance with eccentric training in women with impaired glucose tolerance: a pilot study.' *Journal of Women's Health* 18, 2 (2009): 253–60. doi: 10.1089/jwh.2007.0669

4. Lindberg, E., Benediktsdottir, B., Franklin, K.A., et al., 'Women with symptoms of sleep-disordered breathing are less likely to be diagnosed and treated for sleep apnea than men.' *Sleep Medicine* 35 (2017): 17–22.

   Wimms, A., Woehrle, H., Ketheeswaran, S., Ramanan, D., Armitstead, J., 'Obstructive Sleep Apnea in Women: Specific Issues and Interventions.' *BioMed Research International* (2016). doi: 10.1155/2016/1764837

5. Solano-Pérez, E., Coso, C., Castillo-García, M., Romero-Peralta, S., Lopez-Monzoni, S., Laviña, E., Cano-Pumarega, I., Sánchez-de-la-Torre, M., García-Río, F., Mediano, O., 'Diagnosis and Treatment of Sleep Apnea in Children: A Future Perspective Is Needed.' *Biomedicines* 11, 6 (2023): 1708. https://doi.org/10.3390/biomedicines11061708

   Fernandez-Mendoza, J., He, F., Calhoun, S.L., Vgontzas, A.N., Liao, D., Bixler, E.O., 'Association of Pediatric Obstructive Sleep Apnea With Elevated Blood Pressure and Orthostatic Hypertension in Adolescence.' *JAMA Cardiology* 6, 10 (2021): 1144–51. doi: 10.1001/jamacardio.2021.2003

   Nixon, G.M., Brouillette, R.T., 'Sleep · 8: Paediatric obstructive sleep apnoea.' *Thorax* 60 (2005): 511–16.

6. Westreich, R., Gozlan-Talmor, A., Geva-Robinson, S., Schlaeffer-Yosef, T., Slutsky, T., Chen-Hendel, E., Braiman, D., Sherf, Y., Arotsker, N., Abu-Fraiha, Y., Waldman-Radinsky, L., Maimon, N., 'The presence of snoring as well as its intensity is underreported by women.' *Journal of Clinical Sleep Medicine* 15, 3 (2019): 471–6. https://jcsm.aasm.org/doi/10.5664/jcsm.7678

   Shepertycky, M.R., Banno, K., Kryger, M.H., 'Differences between men and women in the clinical presentation of patients diagnosed with obstructive sleep apnea syndrome.' *Sleep* 28, 3 (2005): 309–14.

7. Young, T., Peppard, P.E., Gottlieb, D.J., 'Epidemiology of obstructive sleep apnea: a population health perspective.' *American Journal of Respiratory and Critical Care Medicine* 165 (2002): 1217–39.

   Young, T., Evans, L., Finn, L., Palta, M., 'Estimation of the clinically diagnosed proportion of sleep apnea syndrome in middle-aged men and women.' *Sleep* 20 (1997): 705–6.

8. Fernandez, R.C., Moore, V.M., Van Ryswyk, E.M., Varcoe, T.J., Rodgers, R.J., March, W.A., Moran, L.J., Avery, J.C., McEvoy, R.D., Davies, M.J., 'Sleep disturbances in women with polycystic ovary syndrome: prevalence, pathophysiology, impact and management strategies.' *Nature and Science of Sleep* 10 (2018): 45–64. doi: 10.2147/NSS.S127475

9. 'How many people in the UK have obstructive sleep apnoea (OSA)?' *Sleep Apnoea Trust* (April 2020), https://sleep-apnoea-trust.org/research/

   Benjafield, A.V., Ayas, N.T., Eastwood, P.R., Heinzer, R., Ip, M.S.M., Morrell, M.J., Nunez, C.M., Patel, S.R., Penzel, T., Pépin, J.L., Peppard, P.E., Sinha, S., Tufik, S., Valentine, K., Malhotra, A., 'Estimation of the global prevalence and burden of obstructive sleep apnoea: a literature-based analysis.' *Lancet Respiratory Medicine* 7, 8 (2019): 687–98. doi: 10.1016/S2213-2600(19)30198-5

10. Courtney, R., 'Breathing retraining in sleep apnoea: a review of approaches and potential mechanisms.' *Sleep Breath* 24, 4 (2020): 1315–25. doi: 10.1007/s11325-020-02013-4

11. Richdale, A.L., Schreck, K.A., 'Sleep problems in autism spectrum disorders: Prevalence, nature, & possible biopsychosocial aetiologies.' *Sleep Medicine Reviews* 13, 6 (2009): 403–11.

    Leader, G., Browne, H., Whelan, S., Cummins, H., Mannion, A., 'Affective problems, gastrointestinal symptoms, sleep problems, and challenging behaviour in children and adolescents with autism spectrum disorder.' *Research in Autism Spectrum Disorders* 92 (2022). https://www.sciencedirect.com/science/article/pii/S1750946722000022

12. Papadopoulos, N., Sciberras, E., Hiscock, H., Williams, K., McGillivray, J., Mihalopoulos, C., Engel, L., Fuller-Tyszkiewicz, M., Bellows, S.T., Marks, D., Howlin, P., Rinehart, N., 'Sleeping sound with autism spectrum disorder (ASD): study protocol for an efficacy randomised controlled trial of a tailored brief behavioural sleep intervention for ASD.' *BMJ Open* 9, 11 (2019): e029767. doi: 10.1136/bmjopen-2019-029767

13. Shaffer-Hudkins, E., Wood-Downie H., Hangauer, J., 'Editorial.' *Child Care in Practice* 29, 1 (2023): 1–2. doi: 10.1080/13575279.2023.2165301

14. Xavier, S.D., 'The relationship between autism spectrum disorder and sleep.' *Sleep Science* 14, 3 (2021): 193–5. doi: 10.5935/1984-0063.20210050

15. Bolic Baric, V., Skuthälla, S., Pettersson, M., Gustafsson, P.A., Kjellberg, A., 'The effectiveness of weighted blankets on sleep and everyday activities – A retrospective follow-up study of children and adults with attention deficit hyperactivity disorder and/or autism spectrum disorder.' *Scandinavian Journal of Occupational Therapy* (2021): 1–11. doi: 10.1080/11038128.2021.1939414

16. Lopez-Leon, S., Wegman-Ostrosky, T., Perelman, C., et al., 'More than 50 long-term effects of COVID-19: a systematic review and meta-analysis.' *Scientific Reports* 11, 1 (2021). https://doi.org/10.1038/s41598-021-95565-8

    Almas, T., Malik, J., Alsubai, A.K., et al., 'Post-acute COVID-19 syndrome and its prolonged effects: an updated systematic review.' *Annals of Medicine and Surgery* 80 (2022).

    Jahrami, H.A., Alhaj, O.A., Humood, A.M., et al., 'Sleep disturbances during the *COVID*-19 pandemic: a systematic review, meta-analysis, and meta-regression.' *Sleep Medicine Reviews* 62 (2022).

    Burns, A.C., Saxena, R., Vetter, C., et al., 'Time spent in outdoor light is associated with mood, sleep, and circadian rhythm-related outcomes: a cross-sectional and longitudinal study in over 400,000 UK Biobank participants.' *Journal of Affective Disorders* 295 (2021): 347–52. doi: 10.1016/j.jad.2021.08.056.

17. Al-Abri, M.A., Al-Yaarubi, S., Said, E.A., 'Circadian Rhythm, Sleep, and Immune Response and the Fight against COVID-19.' *Oman Medical Journal* 38, 2 (2023): e477. doi: 10.5001/omj.2023.38

    Said, E.A., Al-Abri, M.A., Al-Saidi, I., Al-Balushi, M.S., Al-Busaidi, J.Z., Al-Reesi, I., et al., 'Altered blood cytokines, *CD*4 T cells, *NK* and neutrophils in patients with obstructive sleep apnea.' *Immunology Letters* 190 (2017): 272–8.

    Al-Abri, M.A., Al-Yaarubi, S., Said, E.A., 'Circadian Rhythm, Sleep, and Immune Response and the Fight against *COVID*-19.' *Oman Medical Journal* 38, 2 (2023): e477. doi: 10.5001/omj.2023.38

18. Gerritsen, R.J.S., Band, G.P.H., 'Breath of Life: The Respiratory Vagal Stimulation Model of Contemplative Activity.' *Frontiers in Human Neuroscience* 12 (2018): 397. doi: 10.3389/fnhum.2018.00397

    Ledford, H., 'Behavioural training reduces inflammation.' *Nature* (2014). https://doi.org/10.1038/nature.2014.15156

    Kox, M., van Eijk, L.T., Zwaag, J., van den Wildenberg, J., Sweep, F.C., van der Hoeven, J.G., Pickkers, P., 'Voluntary activation of the sympathetic nervous system and attenuation of the innate immune response in humans.' *Proceedings of the National Academy of Sciences of the United States of America* 111, 20 (2014): 7379–84. doi: 10.1073/pnas.1322174111

19. Prather, A.A., Janicki-Deverts, D., Hall, M.H., Cohen, S., 'Behaviorally assessed sleep and susceptibility to the common cold.' *Sleep* 38, 9 (2015): 1353–9.

Cappuccio, F.P., D'Elia, L., Strazzullo, P., Miller, M.A., 'Quantity and quality of sleep and incidence of type 2 diabetes: a systematic review and meta-analysis.' *Diabetes Care* 33 (2010): 414–20.

20. Jackson, E.J., Moreton, A., 'Safety during night shifts: a cross-sectional survey of junior doctors' preparation and practice.' *BMJ Open* 3, 9 (2013): e003567. doi: 10.1136/bmjopen-2013-003567

21. 'Rest breaks at work.' *Gov.uk*, https://www.gov.uk/rest-breaks-work/taking-breaks

22. Blume, C., Garbazza, C., Spitschan, M., 'Effects of light on human circadian rhythms, sleep and mood.' *Somnologie (Berl)* 23, 3 (2019): 147–56. doi: 10.1007/s11818-019-00215-x

    Refinetti, R., 'Circadian rhythmicity of body temperature and metabolism.' *Temperature (Austin)* 7, 4 (2020): 321–62. doi: 10.1080/23328940.2020.1743605

    Refinetti, R., Menaker, M., 'The circadian rhythm of body temperature.' *Physiology and Behavior* 51, 3 (1992): 613–37.

23. Tamaki M., Bang, J.W., Watanabe, T., Sasaki, Y., 'Night Watch in one brain hemisphere during sleep associated with the first-night effect in humans.' *Current Biology* 26, 9 (2016): 1190–4. https://doi.org/10.1016/j.cub.2016.02.063

    Tamaki, M., Nittono, H., Hayashi, M., Hori, T., 'Examination of the first-night effect during the sleep-onset period.' *Sleep* 28 (2005): 195–202.

    Tamaki, M., Nittono, H., Hori, T., 'The first-night effect occurs at the sleep-onset period regardless of the temporal anxiety level in healthy students.' *Sleep Biology Rhythms* 3 (2005): 92–4.

24. Hussain, J., Cohen, M., 'Clinical Effects of Regular Dry Sauna Bathing: A Systematic Review.' *Evidence-Based Complementary and Alternative Medicine* (2018). doi: 10.1155/2018/1857413

25. 'UK adults report poorer sleep, seeing friends less often and exercising less as financial strain takes its toll – new survey results.' *Mental Health Foundation* (17 January 2023), https://www.mentalhealth.org.uk/about-us/news/new-survey-results-report-concerns-due-financial-strain

26. Porcelli, A.J., Delgado, M.R., 'Acute stress modulates risk taking in financial decision making.' *Psychological Science* 20, 3 (2009): 278–83. doi: 10.1111/j.1467-9280.2009.02288.x

    Porcelli, A.J. and Delgado, M.R., 'Stress and Decision Making: Effects on Valuation, Learning, and Risk-taking.' *Current Opinion in Behavioral Sciences* 14 (2017): 33–9.

27. Worley, S.L., 'The Extraordinary Importance of Sleep: The Detrimental Effects of Inadequate Sleep on Health and Public Safety Drive an Explosion of Sleep Research.' *Physical Therapy* 43, 12 (2018): 758–63.

28. Zhang, B., Wing, Y.K., 'Sex differences in insomnia: a meta-analysis.' *Sleep* 29, 1 (2006): 85–93. https://academic.oup.com/sleep/article-lookup/doi/10.1093/sleep/29.1.85

   Mong, J.A., Cusmano, D.M., 'Sex differences in sleep: impact of biological sex and sex steroids.' *Philosophical Transactions of the Royal Society of London Series B, Biological Sciences* 371, 1688 (2016).

29. Mallampalli, M.P., Carter, C.L., 'Exploring sex and gender differences in sleep health: A Society for Women's Health research report.' *Journal of Women's Health* 23, 7 (2014): 553–62. https://pubmed.ncbi.nlm.nih.gov/24956068/

30. Baker, F.C., Sassoon, S.A., Kahan, T., Palaniappan, L., Nicholas, C.L., Trinder, J., Colrain, I.M., 'Perceived poor sleep quality in the absence of polysomno-graphic sleep disturbance in women with severe premenstrual syndrome.' *Journal of Sleep Research* 21, 5 (2012): 535–45. https://pubmed.ncbi.nlm.nih.gov/22417163/

   Nowakowski, S., Meers, J., Heimbach, E., 'Sleep and women's health.' *Sleep Medicine Research* 4, 1 (2013): 1–22. https://pubmed.ncbi.nlm.nih.gov/25688329/

31. 'Sleep and your health.' *Office on Women's Health in the US Department of Health and Human Services* (14 March 2019), https://www.womenshealth.gov/mental-health/good-mental-health/sleep-and-your-health

   Baker, F.C., Lampio, L., Saaresranta, T., Polo-Kantola, P., 'Sleep and sleep disorders in the menopausal transition.' *Sleep Medicine Clinics* 13, 3 (2018): 443–56. https://pubmed.ncbi.nlm.nih.gov/30098758/

32. 'Bloody bedtimes: our survey into the period night-time routines of UK women.' *Bodyform*, https://www.bodyform.co.uk/break-taboos/our-world/bloody-bedtime-routines-campaign/

33. 'Menstrual cycle and sleep.' *Sleep Health Foundation* (24 September 2023), www.sleephealthfoundation.org.au/sleep-topics/menstrual-cycle-and-sleep

34. Jehan, S., Auguste, E., Hussain, M., Pandi-Perumal, S.R., Brzezinski, A., Gupta, R., Attarian, H., Jean-Louis, G., McFarlane, S.I., 'Sleep and Premenstrual Syndrome.' *Journal of Sleep Medicine and Disorders* 3, 5 (2016): 1061.

35. Benca, R.M., Okawa, M., Uchiyama, M., Ozaki, S., Nakajima, T., Shibui, K., Obermeyer, W.H., 'Sleep and mood disorders.' *Sleep Medicine Reviews* 1, 1 (1997): 45–56. doi: 10.1016/s1087-0792(97)90005-8

   Arafa, A., Mahmoud, O., Abu Salem, E., et al., 'Association of sleep duration and insomnia with menstrual symptoms among young women in Upper Egypt.' *Middle East Current Psychiatry* 27, 2 (2020). https://doi.org/10.1186/s43045-019-0011-x

36. 'Menopause and the workplace: How to enable fulfilling working lives: government response.' *Department for Work & Pensions* (18 July 2022), https://

www.gov.uk/government/publications/menopause-and-the-workplace-how-to-enable-fulfilling-working-lives-government-response/menopause-and-the-workplace-how-to-enable-fulfilling-working-lives-government-response

Nelson, H.D., Haney, E., Humphrey, L., et al., 'Management of Menopause-Related Symptoms: Summary.' In: *AHRQ Evidence Report Summaries*. Rockville (*MD*): Agency for Healthcare Research and Quality (*US*); 1998–2005. 120. Available from: https://www.ncbi.nlm.nih.gov/books/NBK11956/

37. Avis, N.E., et al., 'Study of Women's Health Across the Nation. Duration of menopausal vasomotor symptoms over the menopause transition.' *JAMA Internal Medicine* 175, 4 (2015): 531–9.

Baker, F.C., Forouzanfar, F., Goldstone, A., Claudatos, S.A., Javitz, H., Trinder, J., Zambotti, M., 'Changes in heart rate and blood pressure during nocturnal hot flashes associated with and without awakenings.' *Sleep* 42, 11 (2019). https://doi.org/10.1093/sleep/zsz175

38. Baker, F.C., et al., 'Sleep problems during the menopausal transition: prevalence, impact, and management challenges.' *Nature and Science of Sleep* 10 (2018): 73–95.

Kravitz, H.M., et al., 'Sleep during the perimenopause: a SWAN story.' *Obstetrics and Gynecology Clinics of North America* 38, 3 (2011): 567–86.

39. Baker, F.C., et al., 'Sleep problems during the menopausal transition: prevalence, impact, and management challenges.' *Nature and Science of Sleep* 10 (2018): 73–95.

40. 'Hot Flashes.' *The North American Menopause Society*. www.menopause.org/for-women/sexual-health-menopause-online/causes-of-sexual-problems/hot-flashes

'Menopause Strategies: Finding Lasting Answers for Symptoms and Health Trials.' *Fred Hutch Cancer Center*. https://www.fredhutch.org/en/research/divisions/public-health-sciences-division/research/cancer-prevention/msflash.html

41. Elkins, G.R., Fisher, W.I., Johnson, A.K., Carpenter, J.S., Keith, T.Z., 'Clinical hypnosis in the treatment of postmenopausal hot flashes: a randomized controlled trial.' *Menopause* 20, 3 (2013): 291–8. doi: 10.1097/gme.0b013e31826ce3ed

42. Otte, J.L., Carpenter, J.S., Roberts, L., Elkins, G.R., 'Self-Hypnosis for Sleep Disturbances in Menopausal Women.' *Journal of Women's Health* 29, 3 (2020): 461–3. doi: 10.1089/jwh.2020.8327

43. 'Facts and Figures.' *British Heart Foundation*. https://www.bhf.org.uk/what-we-do/news-from-the-bhf/contact-the-press-office/facts-and-figures

44. Cappuccio, F. P., Cooper, D., D'Elia, L, Strazzullo, P., Miller, M.A., 'Sleep duration predicts cardiovascular outcomes: a systematic review and meta-analysis

of prospective studies.' *European Heart Journal* 32, 12 (2011): 1484–92. doi: 10.1093/eurheartj/ehr007

45. Vyazovskiy, V.V., Walton, M.E., Peirson, S.N., Bannerman, D.M., 'Sleep homeostasis, habits and habituation.' *Current Opinion in Neurobiology* 44 (2017): 202–11. doi: 10.1016/j.conb.2017.05.002

    Nagai, M., Hoshide, S., Kario, K., 'Sleep duration as a risk factor for cardiovascular disease- a review of the recent literature'. *Current Cardiology Review* 6, 1 (2010): 54–61. doi: 10.2174/157340310790231635

46. Li, X., Xue, Q., Wang, M., Zhou, T., Ma, H., Heianza Y., Qi, L, 'Adherence to a Healthy Sleep Pattern and Incident Heart Failure: A Prospective Study of 408 802 UK Biobank Participants.' *Circulation* 143, 1 (2020). https://doi.org/10.1161/CIRCULATIONAHA.120.050792

47. Nikbakhtian, S., Reed, A.B., Obika, B.D., Morelli, D., Cunningham, A.C., Aral, M., Plans, D., 'Accelerometer-derived sleep onset timing and cardiovascular disease incidence: a UK Biobank cohort study.' *European Heart Journal* 2, 4 (2021): 658–66. doi: 10.1093/ehjdh/ztab088

48. Scott, H., Lechat, B., Guyett, A., Reynolds, A.C., Lovato, N., Naik, G., Appleton, S., Adams, R., Escourrou, P., Catcheside P., Eckert, D.J., 'Sleep irregularity is associated with hypertension: Findings from over 2 million nights with a large global population sample.' *Hypertension* 80, 5 (2023): 1117–26. https://www.ahajournals.org/doi/abs/10.1161/HYPERTENSIONAHA.122.20513

    Li, C., Shang, S., 'Relationship between Sleep and Hypertension: Findings from the NHANES (2007–2014).' *International Journal of Environmental Research and Public Health* 18, 15 (2021): 7867. doi: 10.3390/ijerph18157867

49. Pinucci, I., Maraone, A., Tarsitani, L., Pasquini, M., 'Insomnia among Cancer Patients in the Real World: Optimising Treatments and Tailored Therapies.' *International Journal of Environmental Research and Public Health* 20, 5 (2023): 3785. doi: 10.3390/ijerph20053785

    Palesh, O.G., Roscoe, J.A., Mustian, K.M., et al., 'Prevalence, demographics, and psychological associations of sleep disruption in patients with cancer: University of Rochester Cancer Center – Community Clinical Oncology Program.' *Journal of Clinical Oncology* 28, 2 (2010): 292–8.

    Savard, J., Morin, C.M., 'Insomnia in the context of cancer: a review of a neglected problem.' *Journal of Clinical Oncology* 19, 3 (2001): 895–908.

50. Montgomery, G.H., Sucala, M., Baum, T., Schnur, J.B., 'Hypnosis for Symptom Control in Cancer Patients at the End-of-Life: A Systematic Review.' *International Journal of Clinical and Experimental Hypnosis* 65, 3 (2017): 296–307. doi: 10.1080/00207144.2017.1314728

    Grégoire, C., Nicolas, H., Bragard, I., et al., 'Efficacy of a hypnosis-based intervention to improve well-being during cancer: a comparison between prostate and breast cancer patients.' *BMC Cancer* 18, 677 (2018). https://doi.org/10.1186/s12885-018-4607-z

51. MacLaughlan, D.S., Salzillo, S., Bowe, P., et al., 'Randomised controlled trial comparing hypnotherapy versus gabapentin for the treatment of hot flashes in breast cancer survivors: a pilot study.' *BMJ Open* 3 (2013): e003138. doi: 10.1136/bmjopen-2013-003138

    Cramer, H., Lauche, R., Paul, A., Langhorst, J., Kümmel, S., Dobos, G.J., 'Hypnosis in Breast Cancer Care: A Systematic Review of Randomized Controlled Trials.' *Integrative Cancer Therapies* 14, 1 (2015): 5–15. doi:10.1177/1534735414550035

52. Chamine, I., Atchley, R., Oken, B.S., 'Hypnosis Intervention Effects on Sleep Outcomes: A Systematic Review.' *Journal of Clinical Sleep Medicine* 14, 2 (2018): 271–83. doi: 10.5664/jcsm.6952

53. Grégoire, C., Faymonville, M.E., Vanhaudenhuyse, A., Jerusalem, G., Willems, S., Bragard, I., 'Randomized, Controlled Trial of an Intervention Combining Self-Care and Self-Hypnosis on Fatigue, Sleep, and Emotional Distress in Posttreatment Cancer Patients: 1-Year Follow-Up.' *International Journal of Clinical and Experimental Hypnosis* 70, 2 (2022): 136–55. doi: 10.1080/00207144.2022.2049973

    Eaton, L.H., Jang, M.K., Jensen, M.P., Pike, K.C., Heitkemper, M.M., Doorenbos, A.Z., 'Hypnosis and relaxation interventions for chronic pain management in cancer survivors: a randomized controlled trial.' *Support Care Cancer* 31, 1 (2022): 50. doi: 10.1007/s00520-022-07498-1

INDEX